Testimonia

"I have always felt the difference between
a great one is their ability to communica   ......g worked with
patients and families in various rehab hospital environments, I've
seen firsthand the powerful effect of compassionate, empathetic
and empowering communication. It makes a tremendous difference in our healthcare system to have effective communicators
with regards to patient outcomes and collaborative efficient teams.
Jennifer has put together a handbook that would be beneficial
for all clinicians and prospective clinicians to read and to guide
their practice every day. I hope it inspires everyone to become
better communicators and thus better clinicians to improve the
quality of our healthcare system as a whole."

—VANESSA ONG-PHYSIOTHERAPIST AND CLINICAL
INSTRUCTIONAL ASSISTANT AT UNIVERSITY OF TORONTO

"Communication is Care provides the unique perspective of
someone who has experienced the healthcare system as the family
member of a patient, but who also understands the challenges of
healthcare providers. As a healthcare provider, it is enlightening
to hear the challenges that a patient and his family underwent.
Those challenging patients we may face as a healthcare providers is likely someone's husband, father, etc. That perspective is
a beautiful reminder that empathy and clear communication
can go a long way in fostering a successful patient-provider
relationship. Communication is Care is a good tool to assist in
self reflection for healthcare professionals. The nine strategies
essentially provide 9 areas in which healthcare professionals can
reflect on and improve in their practice."

—JENNIFER MASSE—PHYSIOTHERAPIST

"Jennifer George's Communication is Care offers nine empowering strategies to assist patients in rehabilitation and health care.
The book combines Jennifer's own personal experiences of her

father's ill health and her experience as a physiotherapist. It provides a heartfelt personal touch and solutions or strategies to assist other healthcare providers in patient care. As a counsellor and coach, I work with clients who require therapist-client rapport first and foremost before any kind of approach, and this book encapsulates the compassionate relationship required in patient care. The book demonstrates heart and soul, as well as a richness to fill the current gaps in health care that sometimes has a tendency to be about the rules and systems rather than about the needs and goals of the patient. I appreciate Jennifer's insights, wisdom, and care in her work, and was truly blessed to have read her book. Thank you, Jennifer."

—LUCY APPADOO—COUNSELLOR AND COACH

"What spoke to me most about this book is how vulnerable the author truly is. Every experience that was shared is a true testament to what she had experienced through her journey. Despite all the noise around her, she chose to take those experiences and put them to a practical use in order to better server her patients. I believe this book is a necessity for not only healthcare professionals, but everyone in all areas of life. The human connection that is emphasized in this book goes much further than a patient-doctor relationship; it embodies true strength and perseverance."

—CRYSTAL SLEIMAN—MARKETING COORDINATOR AND RADIO DJ

"I most enjoyed the personal insights around her father's care and the relationship to and insights brought forward in her own professional practice. The insights shared for integrity and passion, and communication as a key to unlocking healing and establishing an environment to do so is brilliant. Reading about a very personal journey from a family perspective is rare in my field of nursing. Often my interactions are short in the course of a patient's hospital stay, and even more rare would be details after discharge from my care."

—LISA RICE—REGISTERED NURSE AND
REGISTERED MASSAGE THERAPIST

Communication *is* Care

9 EMPOWERING STRATEGIES
TO GUIDE PATIENT HEALING

JENNIFER GEORGE

A Gift for You from the Heart

Visit my website, www.jennifergeorge.co to read
the first three chapters of *Communication is Care: 9
Empowering Strategies to Guide Patient Healing*. You will
also receive ongoing ideas, strategies, and updates about
communication in healthcare.

Let's Stay in Touch

Connect with me on LinkedIN:
https://www.linkedin.com/in/jennifer-george-25656517/

Connect with me on Twitter:
https://twitter.com/jenngeorge08

Enjoy!
~Jennifer

Are you a healthcare provider who wants to go above and beyond, to transform patients' lives? Do you want to be respected as a leader in your field? Can you imagine working with passion and purpose every day despite organizational demands? Do you have a desire to grow professionally?

This is a practical and intuitive guide for current and future healthcare providers who want to communicate with dignity, empathy, and compassion.

Discover how to develop strong communication skills and lead your patients to their highest level of recovery, function, and independence.

In *Communication is Care,* you will find out how to:
1. Define and align your purpose.
2. Practice with compassion and empathy.
3. Listen presently and completely.
4. Guide from a place of integrity.
5. Empower patients to be their own advocates.
6. Focus on solutions, not barriers.
7. Create a safe therapeutic environment.
8. Prevent unnecessary conflict.
9. Reflect and grow with impact.

Jennifer George is a Physiotherapist and was a primary caregiver for more than 10 years. She is transforming the face of healthcare by focusing on communication as the most important tool in patient care. She is a consultant to health professionals and a mentor to students on influential communication in healthcare.

A Note to Readers

This book is for informational purposes only and is not intended as a substitute for the advice and care of your healthcare provider or educator. As with all healthcare advice, please consult with a qualified healthcare provider to make sure this program is appropriate for your individual circumstances. The author and publisher expressly disclaim responsibility for any adverse effects that may result from the application, use or misuse of the information contained in this book.

For information about this title or to order other books and/or electronic media, contact the author:

Jennifer George

www.jennifergeorge.co

jennifergeorge08@gmail.com

ISBN: 978-1-988645-24-7 (print)
         978-1-988645-25-4 (eBook)

Printed in the United States of America

Cover and Interior design: 1106 Design

Quantity discounts and customized versions are available for bulk purchases. For permission requests or quantity discounts, please email jennifergeorge08@gmail.com

Publisher's Cataloging-In-Publication Data
(Prepared by The Donohue Group, Inc.)

Names: George, Jennifer, 1982– author.
Title: Communication is care : 9 empowering strategies to guide patient
      healing / Jennifer George.
Description: [Montréal, Québec] : [Wellness Ink], [2019] | Title from cover. |
      Includes bibliographical references and index.
Identifiers: ISBN 9781988645247 | ISBN 9781988645254 (ebook)
Subjects: LCSH: Medical personnel and patient. | Communication
      in medicine. | Communication in rehabilitation. | Interpersonal
      communication.
Classification: LCC R727.3 .G46 2019 (print) | LCC R727.3 (ebook) | DDC
      610.696--dc23

To Dad

The experiences I have described in this book are based on my memories as a physiotherapist and caregiver. In order to protect the privacy of health care professionals, colleagues, and patients, I have changed some identifying characteristics, places, and details. If any similarities arise, it is purely coincidental.

Table of Contents

Deeply Inspired by…

"And she knew she was a writer. And what writers do is write. They write whether 15 people or 15 million people are reading it. If that is what you believe you are born to do, you do it. You find a way to allow the truth of yourself to express itself. Because that's what we are all looking for—we are all looking for the highest, fullest, expression of ourselves as human beings. And unless you're finding a way for what you believe to be true about yourself to express and manifest itself in the world, you are not living your fullest life."

—*Oprah Winfrey*

Personal Note

It's 5 a.m. on Monday morning. I awake and recite my simple prayer of gratitude. As I get ready to go to the gym, I listen to an inspirational audiobook or podcast to further establish a connection to the world and to myself. My early-morning workouts are another form of gratitude and meditation in motion—a way of honouring my body and mind, which have the ability to function on command and be resilient through the most trying times of my life.

This practice energizes me for what the working week will bring. I pray my patients' weekend went well and wonder about any new patients who may come into my path. I replay the past week in my mind and determine what I will do better, what went well, and what the goals are for the week ahead. I ask myself: how will I bring my best work today? How will I enable my patients to bring their best function today? How will I guide them to start their week on an uplifting note?

I am a Physiotherapist and provide rehab to patients who stay for a prolonged period of time in hospital. In a lot of ways, my patients have lost a sense of their independent identity. They have gone from living life on their terms to living within the framework of the healthcare system—their days are scheduled and regimented according to their medications, personal care, and therapeutic needs.

It is very much like a community. Everyone is here, both staff and patients, for the same purpose: to perform, heal, and grow into our highest, truest selves. In my earlier years of practice, I used to think my success defined who I was. Now I know that it is who I am every day that defines my success and the success of my patients.

And who am I? I am someone who wakes up every morning with the relentless obsession to be my very best—to be in my best health, to love and serve with my best heart, and to leave the best legacy possible. I want to leave this world knowing that I have had a positive impact and that others felt their best when they were around me.

I am grateful to my patients and to my life experiences over the years, as they have taught me so much—to always believe in the greater good, to know that my independence is precious, and to know that we are all deeply connected. No matter how challenging life can get, I now understand there is a higher calling to peace and fulfillment. I realize that the freedom to move, create, and grow is sacred and worth fighting for. Pain, vulnerability, and suffering are what connects all of us, while the shared pursuit of health and happiness keeps us together. If I stop, you stop. If I am fueled, I fuel you. Everybody makes it. That is the way of my world.

I want this book to spark a conversation, a realization, one that triggers mutual feelings of transformation in everyone alike. Whether you are a healthcare provider or a patient, or a healthcare provider who is a patient, I picture you nodding your head as you read line by line of how *communication is the care* given and received every day in our healthcare system. This book embodies all that we are capable of as healthcare providers and all that we are as human beings. Our one, common human denominator is that we are all in *this* together.

Introduction

In 2007, I was 25 years old and finishing my final year of the Master of Physical Therapy program at the University of Western in London, Ontario, Canada. It was during this time that my father suddenly became ill. He was diagnosed with end-stage liver cirrhosis and liver cancer, and he required a liver transplant. He was initially denied the opportunity to be on the transplant list, but, as a family, we pleaded, and, once he had passed the pre-op consults, he was eventually enlisted by the transplant team.

We were incredibly relieved, hopeful, and looked forward to a future with our dad in our lives. We excitedly took the pager from the team and eagerly awaited the call that would determine my dad's fate—the availability of a matching liver. Time was of the essence now; each passing day was unpredictable and increased my dad's risk of becoming sicker. All we had to do now was wait for the call. We prayed and prayed it would come on time.

Eventually the call came, and the hospital had a matching liver. We thought this was the answer to our prayers, the key that would unlock a life of normalcy again. My sister, my mother, and my father drove up to my apartment. They stayed with me, just up the road from the hospital where he would have his surgery. I thought, *This is perfect—my father will have surgery and can recover at my apartment.* Things were starting to make sense again, and the timing could not have been better.

Just days before my father received the call telling him that a matching liver was available, my mother had a spiritually enlightened dream. She dreamt of my late Uncle Lewis, a priest and teacher, sitting under a tree, teaching to five young boys. He then handed my mother a wrinkled, off-white-coloured cloth, and said to give it to my dad. After she noticed it was wrinkled, it flew from her hands like a kite taking flight into the sky.

She then saw another man, a faceless, unknown figure wearing black pants. In his hand, he showed her two livers—one was very vibrant, fresh, and healthy, and the other looked sickly. In her dream, she thought the healthy liver would be my dad's. She interpreted this to be an encouraging dream—reassurance that everything would work out as we believed and imagined.

Although we were grateful, I cannot help but wonder if my dad had a premonition leading up to the surgery. My mom and dad had always been super-intuitively guided by nature. My dad was a man who needed reassurance when it came to most things, especially his health. The day of the surgery, he repeatedly asked the doctors: "Are you sure the liver is good? I don't want to do this again, you know..."

At the time, we did not think anything of it, in fact, we thought he was being funny. A few moments before the surgery, we were informed that the liver was from a donor whose heart was not beating. My dad was asked if he was sure about going through with the surgery. We thought we had no choice. "You always have a choice," the doctor said.

Agreeing to the transplant seemed to be my dad's only hope. He was wheeled into the operating room, pensive and afraid. My dad underwent a liver transplant in February 2007. After the surgery, the surgeon came and told us the liver was a bit tough but that there were no other issues. I remember going to see him in the ICU. My sister gave him the thumbs-up, and he responded with relief in his eyes as he dozed back off. I remember feeling so proud of him—he'd defied the odds of being one of the oldest transplant recipients, attracting medical students to observe his surgery and learn about his story.

Hours passed, and my dad's sleep was getting deeper and deeper, his breathing more laboured. By this time, he had not responded in twenty-four hours. The liver was not taking as we hoped—contrary to my mom's dream but just as my dad had prophesied. Things were starting to spiral as his body was shutting down. The only option was to put him at the top of the nation-wide recipient list for an emergency liver. He basically had twenty-four hours to receive a new liver, or he would die.

Thankfully, a donor heard our weeping prayers. While my dad underwent his second transplant, he was really sick. His bodily organs had all been shutting down, and, by the time he received the second liver, he'd suffered a brain injury and a slew of other chronic health complications. My life forever changed after that moment, and so did his. I never considered that my dad would go into surgery and come out a different man. I never got to say goodbye.

I can recall my mom replaying her dream over and over, thinking to herself, *But your Uncle happily gave me the cloth to give to your dad—how could this be?* Who could have known that the wrinkles would symbolize the lines of suffering my dad would soon endure. For months, his life was supported by mechanical ventilation, dialysis, EEGs, IVs, medications, and catheters. Even long after the machines were detached, his suffering continued.

Where we heard good news, we heard bad news. Where we were trying to hold on, we were questioned as to why. Where we were questioned, we were baffled and unsure. Where we were encouraged, we sought refuge and protection. All of this came from the many healthcare providers we encountered throughout my dad's journey. *One day at a time,* we thought. *One long day at a time.*

After several months in the ICU, the medical team thought it was time for my father to start physiotherapy. I thought that, if I could observe his therapy, it would be great for me to spend time with him and learn from a professional in the field.

I can vividly recall walking into his room: my father was sitting at the side of the bed and the physiotherapist was sitting on a stool in front of him. My dad had a washcloth in his hand, and it was quite obvious that he was confused, agitated, and not following any of the simple commands from the therapist.

I sensed the therapist's frustration as he proceeded to tell me that my father was taking up the majority of his caseload time. He then further challenged me to "think like a therapist and not like his daughter" and asked what I would do in this case.

I took one look at my dad and one look at the therapist and responded, "I *am* thinking like a therapist, and I would continue to work with my patient until I was directed otherwise by the doctors or until his goals were met." My father also responded by throwing the washcloth that he had in his hand out of frustration and protection of his youngest child.

It was in this moment that I made the decision to be a therapist who would lead with empathy, patience, and compassion. After one full year in three different hospitals, my father was discharged. I went on to be his primary caregiver, along with my mother, in our family home, against all odds, for the next ten years of his medically complicated life.

My father passed away in May 2018, and this book is written in his memory and as a tribute for inspiring me to become a healthcare provider who genuinely cares about my patients. Depending on how you see it, I was fortunate to experience both sides of the healthcare system—from the perspective of a caregiver and as a practitioner.

In this book, I have combined eleven years of experience into nine strategies that will guide healthcare providers to communicate with impact and ultimately revolutionize their patients' lives.

1

Define and Align Your Purpose

*M*ost professionals enter into the health-and-wellness industry because they want to positively change lives. As they begin practicing, however, they recognize that the actual amount of time spent directly with patients is quite limited. This is often due to organizational and professional demands, fluctuations in the healthcare system as a whole, and increased patient-to-provider ratios across the board.

As a healthcare provider, you can put only so much energy into each task. By the end of the working day, you feel drained and may even experience a lost sense of self. The majority of studies on health-provider burnout indicate that "…poor well-being, as characterized by depression, anxiety, poor quality of life, stress, and high levels of burnout were found to be significantly associated with more self-reported errors." (Hall, Johnson, et al., 2016).

While I was in my first year of practice, I became a caregiver to my chronically ill father and had uprooted from the city I was living in so that I could move back home and help my mom care for him. During my first few years of entry-level practice, there were some challenging moments where I questioned my calling to serve. The more I was learning about healthcare delivery in its greater form, the more questions I had. I would find myself wondering if I was truly making a difference in people's lives and if there was more that could be done.

One reminder that got me through each day was when my mother asked: "Have you practiced honestly and remained true to yourself and to your patients?" To that, the answer has always been "Absolutely, without a doubt; to help others heal is my purpose for practicing." To that, she would respond, "then you have nothing to fear."

My practice has evolved tremendously over the last eleven years. Whenever I feel stressed, I continue to keep my purpose at the forefront, as it grounds me and connects me to my patients every time. Additionally, I have come to learn and experience that some will support your purpose, some will not, and some will want to see you fail.

And so, it is your obligation to find your way back to your purpose through your own pain even when times feel unbearable and unimaginable. Our purpose is served by us and us alone—no one can give it to us, and no one can take it away. The best way to unite with your purpose every day is to reflect and ask: "Have I practiced honestly and remained true to myself and my patients?" If the answer is "Yes," you have nothing to fear.

The likely reality is that our healthcare system will continue to evolve, change, and expect more from providers in the coming years. However, I have realized that patients are also becoming more aware of these changes and, so, are generally sympathetic to the demands on healthcare providers. The rest is up to us.

Through all of this, patients need to know that *serving their needs is your purpose* during their time with you. If you are out of alignment with your personal and working purpose, it is easily sensed by your patient and will result in poor satisfaction, uncertainty, and hesitation to fully participate in your care.

i) *Defining Your Personal Purpose*

It is not unusual for healthcare providers to feel our health is being compromised because of personal and professional stress. As providers, you cannot look to your patients to bring out your purpose in you, but, rather, you need to bring your purpose to them. We know better than anyone that no one is immune to a stressful life, but you are in a position to help others live better, starting with yourself.

One way to define your purpose is to first take inventory of your own needs. It will be difficult to be in a position to positively change patients' lives if something within is unsettled.

This action to return to peace and harmony within you does not have to be an all-or-none practice but rather a continuous and conscientious journey through life.

First identify what aspect of your own health could be affecting your performance and passion at work. For instance, if physical health is the main concern, it could lead to further physical fatigue and increased risk for injury. Additionally, if the health concern is financial, it could alter the way you perceive your work—is this your "job" or your legacy? Financial stress can impact the passion you put forth every day, and a lack of passion can lead to poor posturing and a drained affect.

Second, you need to find "play" in the process of bettering your health. Reflecting on the simple pleasures that once brought you joy before life got complicated is a good place to start. Implement them as soon as possible, and integrate them into your health plan. For instance, taking the longer commute home from work so that you can blast and sing along to your favourite song on the radio. Or, signing up for a recreational sport that you have not played since high school because life got too busy. A health plan is sustainable if it is flexible, executed with passion, and brings out the best in you. That best part of you will show itself when you begin to feel a harmonious sense of accomplishment and joy with your life.

Once you have identified aspects of your own health to improve upon and have begun to implement the joyful things, it is necessary to find gratitude for the opportunity to do so.

As healthcare providers, you know how fortunate you are to be able to move your bodies on demand, plan your days around your own schedule, eat without difficulty, understand others, and express yourselves clearly.

A sincere word of thanks at the beginning of each day, during the most stressful parts of your day and before retiring at night, can help you to feel empowered, resilient, and satisfied. Gratitude will help to break down the barriers preventing you from achieving self-mastery and fulfillment.

Finding gratitude in the journey is essential because each moment is what matters most. Remember, you are not expected to carry the weight of the world on your shoulders, but *you are* your most important patient. It is ultimately your spirit that will help breathe life back into the lives of your patients. Be grateful for your spirit, protect it, nourish it, and let it touch the lives of others in the way you had always imagined.

ii) *Aligning Your Personal and Professional Purposes*

As mentioned, the healthcare system is continuing to change. More and more people are requiring medical attention, are experiencing complex medical conditions, and are coming from social environments that are quite complicated to return to.

In parallel, healthcare providers' personal lives are also growing more and more complex—many of you have to care for aging parents and younger children, spend more time working to provide for your family or pay off student loans, and feel you have no time to do the things that bring happiness. You may find yourself wondering when your passion to help others started to diminish and how to re-ignite your purpose.

When we have lost a sense of our working purpose, it is often because we feel there is a lack of autonomy, recognition, listening, and support from colleagues and co-workers. It is not the work itself that is the issue—it is the perceived obstacles that prevent us from fully giving ourselves to our work. Furthermore, organizational improvements and changes, although anticipated and appreciated, can take years to actually implement.

Such perceived demands on healthcare providers likely means less time spent with each patient, increased risks to the patient, insufficient resources, more time spent on non-patient care tasks, and minimal opportunity to grow professionally.

However, if you have been committed and consistent to your self-care, you will become more resilient and flexible to workplace stressors. You will find them challenging, not threatening, and be able to manage your stress constructively.

Once you have been begun working at defining your personal purpose, you will eventually be able to flow into your working purpose, as it will become an extension of yourself. This noticeable alignment will result in creating a lasting change in your patients' lives every day and will be noticed by your peers.

If limited time with each patient is the stressor, you will understand it is not the quantity of time that defines your patients' outcomes but, rather, the quality of the care provided during that time. Big leaps can be made with focused treatment and discussion around your patients' goals during each session.

If increased risk to your patient is the stressor, you will better concentrate on your patient's needs and not your own. The care you provide will be governed by compassion and fueled by purpose. You will know there is plenty of time and space for everyone when your patient's safety is of utmost importance.

If insufficient resources are the stressor, you will be able to come up with solutions to facilitate maximal use of the resources available and simply become more creative in providing great care. You will be unafraid to ask for more support, regardless of the response you get, because you know it would best serve your patients and your community.

If administrative tasks are the stressor, you will be efficient at competent documentation while not letting it take more time away from patient care. You will be able to manage your time wisely, always placing greater value on communicating and connecting with your patients, so that the most important aspects of their care are captured and documented.

If lack of opportunity to grow within an organization is the stressor, you will continue to seek ways to improve your personal growth. You will strive to be a leader first in your own life and understand that it is not your title that defines you but, rather, the example you demonstrate every day among patients and team members.

Just imagine your patient or colleague identifying the grace with which you practice and saying to you, "You really love what you do, don't you?" and have it move you magnificently, deeper and deeper into your purpose and overall best being.

iii) Your Purpose Protects

When healthcare providers find our state of "purposeful flow," we become highly sensitive to the negativity and injustices around us. The difference, however, is that you are aware of and personally shielded against the impact of these situations. As you define your personal purpose through pain, you will have nothing to fear because you know the greatest pain is to be in the position of any one of your patients.

And the greatest joy is to free your patients of pain and debility. When you are in a state of flow, you are able to focus in on that one gift that sets you apart from every other provider who deals with the same obstacles. You all have this gift; there may be many healthcare providers in the world who do what you do, but only the purpose-driven touch lives. Why not you?

iv) Your Purpose Matters

Once you have aligned your personal and professional purposes, you live that alignment every single day. It runs so deep that it touches everything you do and all that you are.

Giving care is what you do, but caring is who you are. Healing is what you do, but a healer is who you are. You will exemplify passion in your compassion and recognize that everything you need in order to feel fulfilled is already within you.

Practice with Compassion and Empathy

Once you have established purpose from within, you will be able to intentionally understand the unique needs of your patients. After my father underwent two liver transplants, he lay in bed for months, confused, resistive, and deconditioned.

One evening, I went to visit him, and, although he was disoriented, he was alert. I noticed he had suddenly become incontinent of his bowels, and he was so unsettled from just having soiled himself. I thought to myself, *Is this really happening? How did my father go from a strong, independent man to lying confused in a hospital bed in his own feces?*

Knowing that he could not ask for help, I notified a nurse that he needed assistance. The nurse informed me that she needed another nurse to assist her and that she would come to his room once her partner returned. After much time had passed, I could see my father touching his soiled briefs because he was so uncomfortable and unaware of what was happening. My heart broke for him—I tried my best to just talk to him, calm him, in hopes of distracting him until they returned.

After hesitating for a short while so as not to burden the nurse, I decided to go back and retrieve her because I could no longer watch my dad lie soiled and restless any longer. I knew that he knew what had happened to him, and he was bothered and disappointed by it. I also knew he was trying to clean up his own mess, just as he always did.

At this point, the nurses promptly attended to my dad, and it was difficult for me to watch him be completely dependent on health professionals who truly did not know what kind of man he was before he fell ill. It was all too much to bear in that moment—I remember walking out of the hospital room, crying, and feeling stunned by seeing my fierce father in such a state of helplessness.

The time it took for the staff to attend to my dad made me wonder if they truly understood how it must have felt for him not to be able to independently manage one of his most basic care needs as a human. I also wondered if they really understood how it would feel to be in my position, to witness my father in such a vulnerable state of weakness.

I believe that a compassionate and empathetic connection with your patients begins *before* you directly meet them and is established while reviewing your patients' medical records.

It begins with the intention to put the pieces of your patients' stories together to better understand their needs and how best to facilitate their recovery.

The patients' medical charts are where this process begins. The chart is their *story*, and you are the reader, welcomed into their world and stepping out of your own to imagine what the conditions of their life have been.

By empathizing with your patients' stories, you can then begin to visualize a plan of how you would approach them, proceed with your assessment and care in such a way that validates them, hears their concerns, and positively becomes a part of their next chapter.

Upon meeting with my patients for the first time, I often reference their medical records as a way to guide them in sharing the events of what brought them to my care. I will often ask them if the facts I read, such as dates or medical history, are accurate. If they are, it confirms this with the patients, but on the small chance that they are not, it empowers the patients to share their story correctly from their point of view. My patients' point of view is the one that matters most to me as their healthcare provider. Such intention to understand my patients' perspective helps to fill in any critical gaps and give life to what is written in the consults.

As minimal or as serious as we think our patients' conditions are, all that matters is understanding how our patients perceive and process it. To them, their diagnosis is not just what happened—it has changed their lives. It is important to be mindful and not presume how your patients feel based on how you think *you* would feel.

Once you feel you understand your patients' full story, thoughts, and feelings, you can begin to explain technical aspects of their care in a way that they are able to understand you. Your explanations and recommendations would be tied to what they value most and how you can better help achieve their goals and desires.

As we become experienced and seasoned, it is important not to lose sight of how empathizing with our patients can help heal them through this difficult time. It would be most helpful to combine clinical experience with compassion to intuitively guide patient healing.

For instance, I once worked with an independent-living 85-year-old male who suffered a hip fracture and needed rehab to restore his ability to walk independently. When he first arrived in our care, he lacked confidence and was worried about how he would get back on his feet again. Home was the furthest thing from his mind.

In talking to the patient and learning more about his story, I learned of how strong and independent he was. He was very articulate, social, and carrying out his own care on a daily basis. Yet, he was speaking as though his independence was a distant memory and he was now a different person. However, before he would realize it, through empathy and my experience, I knew he would return home again.

Learning about his story intuitively guided me from one session to the other to build on the things he felt he needed to do to return home. Leading up to his discharge, I asked him to walk with a cane, which he had done before in our sessions, but this would be the first time on his own. Empathetically, I knew he was going to hesitate and be fearful.

Yet, I also knew that he knew he had done this before. He trusted me to try. And he succeeded. Afterwards, he said: "I did not think I could do that on my own, but I knew *you* knew I could. So, I did." He was grateful, he felt confident, and, even better, he met his goal of returning home independently.

The only thing better than being an empathetic healthcare provider is working among a team of compassionate, empathetic providers. For instance, I work with a multi-disciplinary team, and when every discipline is in tune with our patients' sense of being, it is beautiful to witness the evolution of their restored function and independence. To know that every provider played a vital part in our patients' recovery is meaningful beyond words.

This evolution begins from the moment the patients come into the hospital. Generally, patients come to rehab with none of their personal belongings. They are usually received wearing hospital gowns and hospital socks. However, we understand that the moment patients start to feel more like themselves, their desire and level of participation in their care will increase. As such, some of our healthcare providers will often coordinate for patients to have their hair cut or beards trimmed, and arrange for clothing and self-care items with caregivers.

I cannot express how far this goes in the patients' overall outlook on their program, their team of healthcare providers, and their restored sense of self. Since the onset of their admission to hospital, they may actually start to feel like their team cares about them as a human while they work towards their functional needs.

As healthcare providers, we have also been patients at one time or another. Most recently, I had an MRI done on my jaw to determine if I needed surgical intervention.

After I met with my dental surgeon, I then followed up with my family doctor, who had more news to share. During this type of MRI, images of the jaw and brain are taken. At the very end of my MRI report, there was mention of moderate left-sided brain wasting for a woman my age.

The thought of my brain wasting terrified me. All sorts of prognoses were running through my mind, but the provider in me knew to look more rationally. I had no apparent neural signs that would indicate any type of memory loss, personality changes, or movement disorders. At least not right now. My family doctor also helped to explain things compassionately and in a manner *she* would want to hear if the roles were reversed.

A follow-up MRI of my brain was completed, with no concerns. Although I was relieved, I thought to myself, *Imagine a person with no medical background being told that they* may *have a neurological disorder based on a single diagnostic image.* This over-call would naturally provoke fear, worry, and anxiety.

I decided to write this book at the time I found out my brain could be wasting—what a shame that it took a near-life sentence to generate the courage to share my wisdom, truth, and experiences. At any moment, our lives can just shut down, and everything we have been longing to do no longer waits for us.

Life will continue happening around us and beyond us, while we are left wondering how to live again. This book was written with the intention to be more mindful, intentional, and purposeful in my everyday thoughts and actions.

And so, we need to see our patients in their full human form, without judgment, recognizing that the position our patients are in could be any one of us or anyone we care about. In fact, it *will* be you one day. You will find yourself needing service or care from someone in some capacity. I hope you know that the effect your future healthcare providers have on you will affect your ability to cope, your attitude towards your circumstances, and your faith to overcome life's hardships.

Your willingness to simply help your patients demonstrates a genuine connection between you and humanity. I am you, and you are me. The understanding that we are all one helps to gain the trust of your patients and of those in your service.

From now on, when you work with your patients, intentionally communicate with them in a way that you would want others to communicate with your loved ones and yourself—in a way that is dignifying, empathetic, and compassionate.

How to Practice with Compassion and Empathy

Imagine you are just finishing your working day; it was busy, and you are tired. Although your shift is ending, you know that you have a new patient who was just admitted to your care. You are curious to know more but do not want to start a brand-new assessment without being able to fully devote the time your patient needs.

You make a spur-of-the-moment decision to just open your patient's medical chart, and, as you are screening their story, you cannot help but choke up as you see the diagnosis— 30-year-old male with terminal cancer. Suddenly, you realize you have all the time in the world to meet, greet, and begin making your patient feel comfortable in this new environment.

Why? Because you can immediately empathize with your patient's story. From his story, you can imagine the feelings he must be experiencing at such a young age with a terminally defined prognosis. If you were in his place, the last place you would want to be on Earth is in the hospital. However, he has consented to participate because he believes you will help him get to where he really wants to be—in his home, with loved ones, surrounded peacefully as he exits this life.

This situation has happened to me on more than one occasion, and, when it does, I often find these patients have the most pleasant demeanor and zest for life. I always strive to make their sessions with me as enjoyable as possible but often find they put a bigger smile on my face than I do theirs.

They seem to find heartfelt success in the simplest, yet most fundamental, aspects of life that healthier people may take for granted—independently moving in bed, standing up, and taking a couple of steps to move from one surface to another. I know that if I were in such a position, I could care less about the range of motion in my arms and legs, and most about how I can gain enough function to spend precious time with my loved ones.

By taking the time to uncover your patient's story leading up to their illness, you will be better prepared for when you first meet your patient. You will be prepared to understand your patient's feelings, concerns, and challenges as they are expressed to you. You may even develop an image of how your patient may convey this information.

For instance, if your patients have a history of non-compliance, you would try to understand why from their history. During your interaction with them, you would open the channel of communication about what matters most to them. This could give you the insight to communicate in a way that empowers them and creates a sustainable therapeutic relationship. However, if you enter into the interaction with a preconceived notion that nothing you do or say will matter to your patients, you have complicated and terminated the alliance before it has had a chance to succeed.

Empathetic healthcare providers have the ability to clearly explain and educate patients on complexities around their condition and care. This is done with such meaning that your patients feel safe to express themselves, as you are speaking directly to their needs. This does not mean that you have to "dumb things down" or explain things in "layman's terms" for your patients to understand, but it means that you communicate in a way that conveys full attention to your patients' care concerns or questions.

When you are fully attentive to your patients' care needs, you may find yourself being intuitively guided by your patients in providing effective treatment. As a rehabilitative physiotherapist, I am attuned to the fact that patients are striving to reach their maximal level of recovery, function, and independence every single day. By simply empathetically connecting with my patients' day-to-day experiences, I can take in the struggles they are having related to their daily activities and help them work towards overcoming them.

In every treatment session, I look for windows of opportunity to progress patients beyond the day before or even from the beginning of the session to the end. It is not unusual for me to work with a patient who has not stood up in weeks to help them stand after just a short time of working with them. It is also not unusual to spend a full session on walking with a walker or cane because I know that is the one goal that means most to them in that moment.

An empathetic provider might hear feedback from patients, such as: "I did not think I could do it, but you did." You have the ability to be in tune with your patients' emotions and goals, and can competently apply the skills in a way that is unique to each patient. As an empathetic provider, you see not only the sore shoulder—you first see the human being who has a sore shoulder.

As an empathetic provider, you enrich patients' lives. You're not thinking about punch clocks, overtime pay, staffing concerns, or recognition from peers. You are simply and genuinely guided by the intention to serve with compassion in your desire to help your patients.

Although being empathetic can guide and give deeper meaning to your practice each day, you must also be cautious so as not to lose yourself in your patient's journey. Although it is vital to communication and rapport, empathy alone may not heal patients fully. If you become consumed by it, it can potentially result in overstepping therapeutic boundaries and affect your ability to objectively care for your patients.

3

Listen Presently and Completely

Once you have empathized with compassion and have a clearer understanding of your patients as a whole, you can become better aware of their expectations of care and the emotional drivers to participate in your plan.

When healthcare providers first meet with their patients, the rapport is often guided by what is outlined on our assessment forms. While this is helpful to stay organized and may help direct the session, you can become too reliant on it and fail to actively listen to your patients.

By leading with pre-set forms and closed-ended questions, it would be challenging to be fully and completely present with your patients to receive meaningful information and clarify responses. This approach to gathering information, rather than absorbing it, may result in missing critical pieces that could guide the patient's maximal recovery. Human-to-human listening is not one-size-fits-all.

Patient-centered providers are present and completely listen to what matters most to their patients in *that* moment. It requires conscious focus on the verbal and non-verbal messages being expressed, without interruption. To demonstrate you are listening, providers might sit/stand at the level of their patients, make eye contact, nod their head in understanding, or paraphrase in response to their patients' shared information.

Although listening might not formally be a part of your assessment form or therapeutic treatments, it is in the overall practice in which you develop an informative assessment and tailored treatment plan. Sometimes, the practice of listening itself is exactly what your patients need before they can even begin to process participating in your care. It is not unusual to spend the first 10 minutes of a treatment session listening to my patients' concerns or updates before they feel ready to focus on the session's agenda.

In essence, being mindful in this manner can actually minimize your time and stress if your patients are guiding their experience, while feeling fully informed of the risks, consequences, and benefits of participating (or choosing not to) in your care.

Can you recall a time when you first met with your patients and they emotionally started to take your assessment off-course? Perhaps they started to express concern over their children who are too busy to check in on them, or maybe they expressed despair after having lost their spouse just before they fell ill.

It took me a long time to discover that it is in these moments that patient healing begins to occur. Listening to your patients without judging the relevance of their content but, rather, understanding the emotion behind it allows them to feel valued and heard.

This will also allow you to gain a greater understanding of how to encourage, reassure, and motivate your patients. This sense of validation and feeling understood will allow the patient to freely work toward what they seek most from your expertise.

In the same way, when patients are emotionally expressing resistance to participate in your care, it is your obligation to pick up on, listen to, and accept it. In some cases, patients may not verbally express it but, rather, appear frustrated, withdrawn, lack initiative, or seem uninterested.

Healthcare providers should not take personal offence; they should simply ask their patient if it is okay to re-approach them at a later time, if at all. Oftentimes, patients' lack of participation is not a reflection on you but, rather, an expression of something that means more to them than your care services in that moment.

Listening presently and completely to your patients is an ongoing refinement of skill, interaction, and practice. As a clinician, I have experienced on many occasions when my patients felt that they had met their goals, yet I felt that they needed more therapy clinically. Although I thought I knew "best" from a clinical standpoint, my patients knew themselves even better, and I needed to listen to them.

After my father was discharged home in 2008 from hospital, we knew his medical course would continue to be complicated. He had been re-admitted numerous times to the hospital for various infections, seizures, bowel obstructions, and falls. It took an army of us to advocate on his behalf because he was often unable to appropriately verbally answer medical professionals himself.

I can recall too many times over the years when doctors would have a sit-down with our family and explain how medically unwell my father was and that he was likely going to die. Although the medical tests and labs would show he was critically ill, we knew what my father had been through.

These brief hospital visits always paled in comparison to that first visit, when he underwent two liver transplants in 2007 and came out a different man. Although we knew that, many providers did not fully listen to the story of his undying spirit.

We were at such a high risk for burnout that many professionals could not understand how we coped and managed. But we knew my dad. The hospital environment often confused my dad—it was not his home—he was always disoriented, resistant to care, and wanted only his family by his side, especially my mother. We felt we were at greater risk for burnout while he was in hospital because we always had to be there to provide care, as he could be so resistant to staff.

Despite how medically unwell he seemed to doctors, he was more stable at home than in hospital. Home is where he thrived. We always advocated for him to be discharged the moment he was medically stable enough to do so, even if he had not walked in days, because we knew that when he returned home, things would click for him again. And they usually did.

I have learned from being a caregiver that patients' satisfaction and level of participation would be much improved if the purpose of the interactions were focused around what they ultimately desire. For instance, if patients express that they are content with their treatment outcomes and wish to pursue a different path to support further healing, then it is our duty to listen, plan the follow-up to their discharge, and remove our egos from the equation in the process.

When I was working through my Master's, I can recall being given very little insight into the importance of communication in healthcare. Many programs currently do not completely recognize that communication is fundamental to patient care and clinical-skill application. Through my research, I have had great difficulty finding evidence to support that teaching provider-patient communication skills is happening among professional students.

Much of the research shows a need for it to improve the quality of patient care and experiences. Some authors have even established their own post-grad courses, but there is no concrete evidence to support that this learning is in fact happening in health-professional schools *across the globe.*

Perhaps organizers believe that communication is a skill naturally embedded in students and that, if they'd reached this level of academics, they can inevitably communicate in a manner that optimizes patient outcomes. Or, perhaps it is too vast a topic to teach and too difficult to narrow the focus for a complete curriculum.

What organizers may fail to realize, though, is that our world is changing and is becoming more dominated by artificial intelligence and technology. As such, human-centered communication is needed now more than ever. Patients are often vulnerable, as they have lost a sense of independence and control over their lives, and so, if a solid provider-patient rapport cannot *first* be established, then the delivery of other aspects of care will always fall short.

Imagine if professional institutions had at least one clinical placement where students would not focus on the technical or clinical skills but solely on the communication between their preceptor and patients. Six weeks of real-life, human-to-human, provider-patient observation. This would greatly enhance the skill of listening presently and completely in the future healthcare provider.

Not only will the students gain a greater understanding of the value communication has in patients' outcomes and satisfaction, but perhaps we as providers could even learn from our students. Communication will continue to evolve, just as our healthcare system and clinical skills do. This deserves to be further researched and examined—don't you think?

From years of reflecting and asking myself, "Why did patient A improve, and why did patient B fall short?" I have come to realize that communication *is* the care we provide to patients. Communication is why patients with similar impairments and similar treatment approaches never experience the same results. It is not just a soft skill—it is core to all other skills.

Ultimately, most of us can learn clinical skills with consistent review, practice, and patience. Yet, becoming the healthcare provider in unforeseen circumstances—those in which your patient does not fit into the checkboxes on those forms—can be magical when you remain present, listen completely, and individualize the plan according to your patient's needs at that time.

How to Listen Presently and Completely

Upon graduating, I can recall being very ambitious and eager to develop my clinical skills. I invested so much of my time and finances into post-graduate certifications because I believed that is what would produce the best results for my patients. After all, foundational knowledge, clinical skills, and safe patient handling were the primary focus of every class.

While this was absolutely necessary and prepared me for entry-level practice, I now realize that there was not enough emphasis on communication development and rapport between healthcare providers and patients. Although possessing and developing clinical-skill competencies is a professional requirement and can enhance patient outcomes, if they are not implemented according to your patient's goals or needs, they can have minimal effect or no effect, or even cause harm.

While it is always essential to have a variety of skills to treat patients with different clinical impairments, many of us can be too concerned with being "right" and outputting skill rather than taking in our patients' feelings, experiences, and perspectives. While it is important to be competent at diagnosing and treating, neither will be effective if we are not competently communicating the delivery and listening to the response.

A study on the nature of patient complaints by Raberus et al. (2018) demonstrated that "communication needs to be improved overall" and that "patient vulnerability could be successfully reduced with a strong interpersonal focus." In addition, Reader et al. (2014) discovered through their systematic review on patient complaints in healthcare that treatment and communication were the most common.

Perhaps if healthcare providers and organizational leaders recognized that communication is care, it would get just as much training and skill development as clinical-treatment application. As a result, interpersonal-communication skills among providers would improve, and fewer patient complaints would occur globally. This investment could save the healthcare system from losing money as it could reduce patient length of stay, patient injury, and malpractice suits.

As health professionals, achieving licensing in our chosen field is competitive in nature, as there is a minimum academic grade that must be met in order to be accepted into educational programs. It has been my experience through school and in employment that a competitive mindset persists within us beyond graduation, a self-inflicted pressure which continues to revolve around being everything to everyone. This is not limited to your patients and caregivers but extends also to your own loved ones.

As such, it may be more difficult for healthcare providers to reach a point of mindfulness in our practice—being aware of and letting go of the ideas and anxieties that are constantly on our mind to allow ourselves to be fully present in our patients' presence. If we are constantly outputting information, even if only in our minds, this can create a block to accurately receiving the verbal and non-verbal expressions from our patients.

You may think you are giving your patient your full attention simply because you are working one-on-one, however, if your patient cannot follow because you are preoccupied and overtly running around in your mind, you will lose your patient's interest and trust instantly.

Remember, patients are well aware of the demands on healthcare providers. They understand that we serve many others in addition to them, however, when our patients are in our care, it is expected that our focus is on their concerns, not the other way around.

One part of listening is asking questions to learn more about your patients. This demonstrates that you take a genuine interest in who they are. Listening to your patient's story and history can often add value in coming up with collaborative goals and an individualized plan.

For instance, some physicians go above and beyond with their approach to patients by literally sitting in a chair by their patients' bedside and conversing with them about their history, current state, and goals. This approachable posturing is critical to the patients' sense of ease, importance, and value.

When we ask patients questions about their health journey, it helps us to gain a better understanding of what they were like before they fell ill and where they feel they need to be to regain function and control over their lives again. Keep in mind that this process is *ongoing*. You need to be constantly listening to your patients in every session, as it may spark that one intervention that is unique to their needs and will propel them one step closer to their goals.

Other ways of listening presently and completely to your patients include maintaining eye contact and not looking at your watch or clock in the room, nodding your head as a gesture of understanding and eagerness to learn more, and rephrasing your patients' words in a way that highlights how it could be affecting the way they feel currently.

If a patient appears to be highly confused or incapable of making informed decisions, it is our responsibility to call upon the patient's substitute decision-maker to fill in any gaps we may be experiencing. By involving our patients and their caregivers or family, it may further improve patients' trust in us, even if they cannot express it directly.

For example, if you are working in long-term care facilities among residents with significant cognitive deficits, it is important for you to "listen" and take note of what the residents' routines and interests are and be creative with timing and treatment.

I can recall working with a resident who had severe dementia and would chronically clean on the unit. In order to maintain her attention for more than five minutes, her treatment plan was integrated into her cleaning routine. This allowed her to engage in human interaction, improve her functional mobility, and maintain participation in her day-to-day living.

You may also be met with patients who have difficulty coping with the seriousness of their medical status or feeling debilitated by their pain. Your patients could be having difficulty imagining themselves functionally improving to a level of independence.

You will need you to hear them out, validate their feelings, and educate them on your experience and how you plan to help them progress toward their goals. This will need to happen repeatedly until you and your patient are on the same page of communication and treatment progression.

Even when we think we know exactly what it is our patients need to restore their health and vitality, our patients may be able to tolerate it only in small doses. We may think we know one day but can soon find ourselves way off the next day. Which is why we must always be present to meet our patients where they are at and gain their trust in every interaction in order to help them move onward. This takes time to evolve, to truly tune into what your patients are saying, especially when they have nothing to say.

4

Guide from a Place of Integrity

"Integrity," as a whole, can be complex and can mean different things to different people. It has been defined as "what you do when nobody else is around, or what you do and how you do it on a daily basis. Integrity means our actions are honest and trustworthy" (Healthcare Compliance Pros, 2018).

As healthcare providers, our integrity is what genuinely guides us to deliver high-quality, ethical, and fair care to our patients. We all have those days where it is non-stop, putting out one fire after another, but in the midst of all of this, you know that you are maintaining excellent care by acting in the best interests of your patients.

It was August 3, 2007, my birthday and six months after my father's liver transplants. He was being discharged from one hospital and transported to another hospital, which was a long drive away. Accordingly, my family and I drove our own vehicles and expected to meet my dad at the new hospital. When we arrived, my father and the transport van were nowhere to be found.

We waited and grew more and more concerned. Phone calls were made, and we learned that, apparently, part way through the ride, my dad had become highly agitated, and they needed to return him back to the primary hospital. While we understood the circumstances, we could not understand why we were not informed that he was back at the hospital while we were all driving away. It seemed only logical and responsible to inform us, instead of us being left to put the pieces together on our own.

In short, my sister and I drove all the way back to the hospital, and when we arrived at the floor, we could hear my father screaming out at us: "Hey! Heeeey! Over here!" He sounded angry, restless, and distressed. He was sitting on a big reclining chair by the nurse's desk, which is a common practice for staff to keep an eye on agitated patients. As he was calling for our attention, he was slamming his hand down on the lap tray that restrained him. My heart broke for him, for all of us.

Knowing my mother was by his bedside for a minimum of sixteen hours a day, seven days a week, did the hospital staff consider how it might make my dad feel alone? Was there even a thought given to how our family would feel driving, exhausted, expecting to meet our dad at the new hospital to ease his transition?

As a healthcare provider, I cannot imagine not informing family of such an eventful circumstance in their loved one's care, as it would only create more stress on my patient and the family—not to mention the unnecessary stress for me to have to handle their concerns. Although my dad was one of the most challenging patients I had ever come across, he'd always been a little bit better with his family by his side, and his team of providers knew this.

There are no right or wrong answers, as everyone's sense of integrity is different. Some might not have been as impacted by the lack of communication as we were. However, this was a traumatic event for me, one I will never forget. The perceived lack of care left an imprint on me and my future practice. When I communicate with patients, I try my best not to leave any loose ends. If circumstances around my patients' care change, patients or other family are the first to be informed.

When you make the decision to be a health professional, it is because you have an inner desire to reliably lead others to optimal wellness and function. It is not to say that you should lead from a bold, extroverted, and authoritative position but, rather, genuinely lead by example each day.

I once was in a treatment space with a patient who was communicating with my colleague. I am not sure of what exactly transpired between them, but I vividly remember the patient abruptly and bluntly stating: "How do you expect me to take advice from you when you do not look the part of physiotherapy?"

While it seemed apparent that the patient was focusing solely on my colleague's outer appearance, I think she was referring also to her general demeanor. My colleague appeared stressed, uncertain of herself, and perhaps lacking her own form of self-care.

While the patient could have been politer about what she said, she was essentially pointing out that the provider was not "walking the talk" and was therefore, felt to be unreliable in taking on her care needs.

Integrity is also demonstrated throughout our day-to-day interactions and communicative practices. Patients can sense if you practice with integrity by simply observing how you handle their care and the care of others.

Are you trustworthy? Will you follow up when you say you will? Will you keep them informed? Can you work with the rest of the team to handle your patients' concerns or questions? How many times can you recall your patients saying that they had test X Y Z done months ago but never heard back? How many times have patients told you their family member has questions about their care? How many times have you heard the call bell ringing endlessly while you were standing outside of the patient's room?

I remember bringing a new patient to the rehab gym for her first day of treatment. I asked her how she was feeling, and she abruptly responded, "I feel mixed up." I asked her to elaborate, and she went on to mention how she had no idea as to what was going on with her care, how she felt she had too many providers who were not communicating with each other; she was wondering how she even ended up in our facility.

After I listened to her concerns and validated them, she consented to participate in the assessment. She had questions during our session that only the doctor could answer. I made it a point to tell her that I would personally leave the doctor a message to follow up with her concerns directly.

Later that day, I followed up with her to confirm if the doctor had seen her. Sure enough, he had and was attentive to her questions. After that moment, I found her demeanor to be much more upbeat, and she was more engaged in her treatment plan every day.

If you want your patients to trust you and believe in your competency as a leader, then you must follow up on their concerns. Even if you are not qualified to answer their questions or provide the specific care needed, then connect them as soon as you can to the provider who can help.

It is these minimally demanding but highly effective interactions of integrity that help put your patients at ease, improve their compliance in your care, and allow them to focus on the goals of their treatment.

Integrity is a core value of every human being. We all want our concerns addressed. Do not wait for someone else to handle the follow-up, because that is what everyone *else* is doing—they are waiting for the next provider and then the next provider—and nothing changes. Be the provider who sets the bar and creates change by demonstrating action. Restore your patients' faith in the system and in the goodness of humanity.

To guide with integrity also means that you completely believe in your philosophy and practice it every day. This is demonstrated in your character—do you value health and vitality? Would you practice the very education and techniques you share with your patients? Can you relate to your patient on a mutual level of functional achievement? Do you value communication as care?

Fundamentally, if we are treating a health concern of our patients, we would be expected to be in pursuit of our own health goals or already be of sound physical, emotional, spiritual, or mental health. Otherwise, how can you expect your patients to follow your lead if you are unable to first lead yourselves? Your personal integrity strengthens the connection with your patients as it shows the humanistic side of bringing your best health and work every day.

Experience aside, as I reflect on my own personal practice over the years, I know I am a better practitioner today than I was in the first six years of my career. During those first few years, I was active but unfit, uninspired, super stressed, and unclear as to which direction I wanted to focus on professionally. It was not until I decided to make my own health and well-being a priority that my self-belief and impact on my patients significantly improved.

As a physiotherapist, I have had the remarkable opportunity to work in many different environments. With each passing year of my practice, I felt I was getting closer to the workplace that shared the same values as myself. Although I learned some hard lessons along the way, I held onto and demonstrated the belief that there was an organization out there that upheld similar values in delivering outstanding patient care and teamwork.

After six years of practice, I took a chance on a casual position that would allow me to progress and restore patients' function. At that point, the thought of working fewer hours and making less income was worth the valuable experience and impact I could have on changing a few people's lives. I am incredibly grateful to say that I am still with this organization today and revolutionizing patients' lives full-time.

As healthcare providers, we do not need to be perfect in every aspect of our own health, but we need to be able to relate to and lead our patients by example. Everyone has a different journey when it comes to our personal health goals, but we should be on a journey of health nonetheless and be dedicated to it. Your patients will feel reassured knowing that, if you have your best health at heart, you will have theirs, too.

How to Guide with Integrity

As healthcare providers with integrity, we essentially guide patients by our ethical standards. In order to determine your standards for delivering care, you should first reflect on the values that matter most to you in your personal life and in your practice. You should then align yourself with an employer or organization who upholds the same standards and supports you to practice with excellence every day.

Looking back, when I was an entry-level physiotherapist, I tried to fit into the framework of some of my previous workplaces. I always loved helping others to achieve their highest level of function and deeply believed in my patient-care philosophies. However, when I felt limited by employers or organizations in delivering quality care ethically, it began to interfere with my passion and resulted in poor workplace satisfaction.

When you are an entry-level provider, it is natural to trust that employers have your best interests at heart and, even more importantly, value high-quality patient care above all else, just as you do. This naiveté comes from the pure intention of just wanting to help others and not understanding that there is a bigger business or organizational framework that is supposed to support you in doing so.

In my earlier years of practice, I conflicted with organizations that, due to financial reasons, did not allow me to build rapport and provide excellent service to my patients. In my mind, it just did not and still does not make sense. While I know that business is business, good health is priceless.

As far as I was concerned, if a patient needed therapy, they needed therapy, and I was not going to let something like money or time stand in my way. That is what I believed, and I always held on to that, no matter how many times employers tried to slap my hands for not generating enough revenue.

Whenever I realized my values were out of alignment with an organization's and there was no way of coming to a working agreement, I resigned without regret (even if it took me longer to recognize). I now know that I cannot assume that others uphold the same moral standards as I do. If I do not practice what I believe to be in the best interests of my patients, no one will ever believe in my values, and no one will support or try to understand my work.

Once I realized it was me, my standards, and my moral right and responsibility to practice them despite disagreement, then opportunities started coming into my path. This resulted in soaring patient outcomes and workplace satisfaction. This is where I am today and, through this book, is how I continue to evolve. My hope is that healthcare providers begin to grow together and move our professions forward in positively impacting people's lives.

In today's world of social media advertising and marketing, there are many health professionals who disrespect other professionals, whether indirectly or directly, to attract clientele and boost their presence. If I were a patient, I would feel conflicted by this—is this healthcare provider truly looking out for my well-being? Why are they hurting others if their purpose is to serve and help people? This is completely the opposite of what having integrity means, as it shows a complete disregard for your peers and profession.

Growing up, I was always the encourager, the one who rooted for the underdog. I always believed everyone could make it. People used to see this trait in me as being inspiring, strange, and even funny at times. I never knew how to be any other way—it was just who I was. Now I realize that it is my unique gift to my profession, patients, and personal relationships.

If you believe there is a bigger purpose to your work, you have to believe in it through the good and the not-so-good. You should never settle for a position that resists professional growth, minimizes or streamlines your skills and abilities, and places profit over patient care. This may take time to develop as you gain life and work experience, but know that there will always be a more ethical opportunity that supports your moral agreements.

In addition, if you are a provider who works in a multidisciplinary team, it is important to develop a strong rapport with your colleagues and strive to collectively produce the best patient experiences. Communicate with each other and demonstrate to patients and caregivers that the whole team is part of their health solutions. This will boost patient-to-provider trust and demonstrate genuine concern for your patients. It will also improve workplace satisfaction by giving everyone a sense of belonging, one in which team members help each other out through challenging moments and recognize each other during the successful ones.

The old saying "Success is a lonely road..." does not really apply to the healthcare provider. Healthcare providers with integrity realize they are only one piece of their patients' puzzle to success and that unity of the providers amplifies the success of their patients.

Imagine the global impact this could have if we communicated fluidly with each other, rather than just territorially focused on our own scope. We all have a part to play, and, while our patients are the key players, their success is built on the foundation of the wall of providers that surrounds them and fosters their growth.

During your lifetime as a healthcare provider, you will also need to feel supported, as you are constantly caring for others. It is often your colleagues who best understand the beauty of delivering remarkable patient care that leaves you feeling proud, even at the expense of your sleep or risk for injury. If you are tired by the end of each working day and find yourself reflecting on what went well and what you would do better, then you are doing something right. You are living with integrity.

I challenge you not to look at your work as only your job or career but as your legacy. Helping others is a part of who you are, not just part of what you do. By living with integrity, you are living your legacy. You will be recognized not only for being competently skilled at what you do but also for being an anchor of encouragement and support when your patients need it most.

As you practice with integrity, you will recognize that healthcare is not only a *reliable* profession—one that will pay well and provide ample opportunities—but that it is also one of the most *trusted* professions. And you are being trusted to do what is right for your patients every day, in the face of adversities.

While that comes with great responsibility and risk, it is also comes with high reward. It will tire you, it will challenge you, it will strengthen you, it will fulfil you, and it will humble you to your knees. It will humanize you. It will give your life more meaning as you pour meaning back into the life of your patients.

5

Empower Patients to Be Their Own Advocates

"Dear God, please keep my parents happy and healthy. Thank you for allowing them to be a part of my life for this long." Every night before falling asleep, I'd utter this simple prayer. It was 2006, the year before my dad's liver transplants, and I was preparing to move away to complete my Master's. My parents were older than the average parents with children my age. They remained independent deep into their 60s, and I always tried to be mindful and appreciative of the time spent with them.

Later into the middle of that night, I was awoken by the sound of my father vomiting. I thought it was a side effect of the antibiotic he'd been prescribed earlier that day for a throat infection. I knew it was more when I heard my mother's concern: "What is this? What's going on?!" I got out of bed and walked into the bathroom, where my father stood, hunched over in front of the toilet, with my mother by his side supporting him as copious amounts of blood were uncontrollably projecting from his mouth.

It looked like a murder scene—blood splattered and smeared all over the walls. I thought I was going to faint, and I started to head back to my room, but as I walked by my father's room, I could not help but notice the clots of blood all over his pure white sheets. This would mark the beginning of my father's health journey and our relentless advocacy as a family.

After this episode, he was in and out of the hospital to manage similar hemorrhaging that happened on multiple occasions. However, it was after the third episode that my father was diagnosed with liver cancer and was informed that his only treatment option was a complete liver transplant. My father's medical team was reluctant to put him on the transplant list because he was older than the recommended candidates, and so a lot more risk would be involved.

As the team was informing us of this, we were all gathered together in the conference room. My father felt defeated and hopeless. With his delicate hands clasped in a prayer-like fashion, resting on his lap, looking down, he stated, "So you're just going to send me home with cancer?"

Our family begged and pleaded for the transplant team to put my father on the list, as he was getting more and more sick, so any surgical risk would be worth saving his life. It was not until his fourth hemorrhage that the team finally accepted our pleas and put my father on the transplant list.

Just imagine that, one day you are living life, free, independent, and happy, and then you are suddenly derailed by an illness that has you requiring medical care. The next thing you know: you are in a cold, lit room, lying on the thin mattress of a hospital bed, and you can feel the uncomfortable bed frame beneath you. You are wearing a hospital gown, covered by a thin white sheet and crisp blanket, wondering, *How did I get here?*

All you know is that you need medical care but are uncertain of how the system works. You meet multiple well-intentioned people who are there to help, yet you cannot remember a single one of their names. You just feel like you have no control over the course of events that are about to take place. Things might feel like they are beginning to spiral. What do you hold on to?

Choice. Hope. It is difficult to feel like you have choices and hope when you suddenly have to rely on medical experts to look after your health as you try to learn what has happened to you.

As healthcare providers of integrity who are empathetic and present with your patients, one of the best ways to improve care is to empower them to be involved and make choices around their health goals. Whether the options are good, bad, or worse, the freedom to choose in one of the darkest moments of their lives will help build trust and rapport.

Every interaction should be an opportunity for patients to present any concerns, questions, or feelings, and be fully educated about the care around their needs. Whether the prognosis is favourable or not, patients and caregivers will always be grateful for the opportunity to direct their care while feeling fully informed along the way.

While your patients understand that you are doing the best you can to provide the highest quality of care possible, they need to feel like they are a part of their team, too. This is their life, their body, their mind, their faith, their joy, their peace, their choice. Your goal is to empower and facilitate them to make the most informed decision possible, one that they can live with and one that they feel they have made for themselves.

I have worked with many patients over the years, and, while we did not always see eye to eye on the recommended plan, their compliance and trust in me as their provider was always greater when they had the final say in their treatment or discharge plan. As their healthcare provider, my role is to offer my expertise around what is recommended, while explaining the risks, benefits, and consequences.

In such circumstances, I find myself open to what my patients' thought processes are. Sometimes I learn something new from them that could help another patient, or they gain a new perspective on how to better treat and manage their conditions. My aim is always to find the safest way to support my patients' choices. A common example of this occurs in hospital or in long-term care facilities, where I would recommend patients to call for assistance when they want to get out of bed because of balance or strength issues, but they intentionally refuse to do so.

Although they are well aware of the risks of not following through with what is recommended, I am still committed and obligated to support their decision by making suggestions to make their environment safer.

For some, this might mean using a bed alarm, if the patient is agreeable. In some cases, patients feel restrained and institutionalized by the idea of alarms, and so, again, we go back to the drawing board to empower them but still reduce their risk of falling. Sometimes patients will choose the risk of falling over feeling reliant on others. Although I could never understand that, who am I to judge?

Other common examples include patients choosing to return to work or social environments that put them at high risk for re-injury or readmission to hospital. There is no worse feeling than helping patients to restore their function and regain independence while knowing, in the pit of your stomach, you will see them again. I make peace with myself by knowing I have said and done all that I could to make their lives a little safer than before.

In some cases, part of empowering patients to be their own advocates is giving them the opportunity to choose their healthcare provider. There is nothing wrong with saying to yourself, "I know someone who can help my patient better than I can" and offering this choice to your peer and patient. This in itself is providing quality care and is one of the highest forms of knowing oneself—acknowledging both your strengths and your limitations.

Empowering patients to be their own advocates can be emotionally demanding on healthcare providers. This is because you know some patients are choosing to live at a level of risk you do not recommend and that they may lack the insight or concern to notice. In such cases, I recommend you circle back to your care team, ask for help, guidance, and a clearer understanding. Do not become all-consumed by the choices you do not agree with, but do not give up too easily, either.

You will better be able to cope by the end of the day knowing you have done your best and knowing that your patients were still grateful for your care. Take your ego out of it, as your patients' journeys are never about you. You will always have many patients who are eagerly looking to you for safe guidance toward the next step in their care plan.

In the event that a patient is cognitively confused and unable to make their own decisions, healthcare providers can communicate with the patient's family to help come up with the best plan of care.

Once my father had received and survived the second liver transplant in February 2007, he suffered a brain injury. The surgical healing was suddenly compounded with an even greater problem: his altered state of mind. He was delirious, confused, and disoriented. He was also lacking the ability to breathe, speak, eat, move, sit, or stand on his own for a whole year.

In fact, his frontal lobe had been severely affected. The frontal lobe occupies two-thirds of the human brain and governs high-level cognitive functions, attention, memory, and language. It also processes mood, personality, and reasoning (Chayer, Freedman, 2001).

In September of 2007, my father was finally discharged home for the first time. The discharge seemed too early, as he was still medically unwell—he had been vomiting, he was weakening, and he was disoriented. It was just a couple of weeks later that he was readmitted to the hospital again, on Thanksgiving Day.

This resulted in another prolonged hospital stay, and it seemed as though things went from bad to worse. The focus appeared to be more on his neurological state than the rest of his body's healing. No one seemed to really consider his full history—a 69-year-old man who had undergone two liver transplants within one week of each other and, on top of that, had suffered a brain injury.

In fact, one of the most disheartening situations had occurred during this time. The doctor who had been overseeing my father's care appeared to be either at a loss or unconcerned about his circumstances. She had placed the onus on us, the family, as "forcing" my father to live.

She had expressed that "there was the force of nature, and then there's the force of the family." She went on to say that his brain was more than "50% gone" and then, in the same breath, turned to my just-deemed-incapable father and asked if he wanted to live this way, lacking independence.

My father did not respond to her question and instead told her he did not like her. The doctor abruptly left, stating my father was not well. Little did she know that he was medically unwell but very much alive. It was our role as my father's advocates to *make* professionals realize he was still worth caring for and not *assume* that they would recognize that he was.

As a healthcare provider and a caregiver, I understand that doctors and other professionals who are able to give a prognosis will have to give unwanted news. That is, unfortunately, part of their position. The problem here, however, is that this doctor failed to give us any news, any medical reasoning, and the manner in which it was proposed was downright uncompassionate.

We felt that there were still medical needs that had to be resolved before a reasonable discharge plan could be put in place. We had contacted patient advocacy and the doctor, but the doctor hung up on us, and, unfortunately, nothing changed through patient advocacy.

As a family, as his caregiver, I felt that we were being recognized as a barrier rather than a facilitator to my father's care. We felt we were being excluded and that care-plan decisions were being presumed without our consent and input. Although my father could not follow direction from professionals at the time, he trusted we would advocate for him.

We knew him better than anyone else did on paper. We understood that my father's medical situation was extremely unique, complex, and challenging. Yet, rather than using us to help guide his case, we were being made to feel problematic because we were advocating for the best care possible.

Eventually, we advocated for another doctor, and she instantly developed a positive rapport with my father. It did not change how sick my father was, but at least we all felt at peace communicating with a provider who empowered us to advocate for my father's care needs.

This experience with my dad made me realize that every moment a provider-patient interaction occurs, the patient is advocating for their needs, concerns, complaints, and goals. As providers, we need to encourage patients to be forthcoming and not let the provider assume the patients' intentions of participating in our care. It is more challenging to work with a patient who is flat and uninvested than it is to work with a patient who wants to feel better and is aware of their potential.

I can recall many times over the years where patients felt they were more independent in their mobility than I did. In such moments, I was fully transparent with the patients about the risks and consequences of their decisions from a provider standpoint. In some cases, patients understood the risks and were agreeable to the recommendations. In other cases, patients understood the risks and did not follow through on my recommendations.

In the event that patients do not follow through and you know they are living or moving at risk, it is best to come up with a supportive plan to minimize their risks. You can also refer or involve other healthcare providers who can further support your patients' decisions and ease them into a safe transition. Patients need choices in order to feel a sense of control over their lives again. Provide your patient with the best suggestions—the ones that minimize their risk of injury or harm.

How to Empower Patients and Caregivers to Be Their Own Advocates

One of the most valuable tools to empower your patients and caregivers to be their own advocates of care is to ask for permission. From the moment you introduce yourself, to every interaction thereafter, ask for their permission to discuss their history and share their concerns, goals, and expectations. Additionally, ask for their permission to provide direct care during every interaction.

By asking your patient for permission to interact and work with you, you are taking away the self-perceived burden some patients feel they have placed on you. This will give the patient the opportunity to feel like you not only *have* to provide care but that you *want* to provide care and help them.

Another way to empower your patients and caregivers to be their own advocates is to give them the freedom to choose the path to their goals. By offering your patients more than one method to best achieve their desired outcomes, you are being adaptable and attentive to their individual needs. Give your patients choices; empower them to choose the solutions that are right for them; present yourself as a collaborative partner and not the authority over their life.

Empowering your patients to be their own advocates is essentially conveying that your goals are your patients' goals. If you foresee an inability to achieve their goals, then having an honest and straightforward discussion would help your patient to re-establish new goals and empower them to take charge of the circumstances around their desired outcomes.

As healthcare providers, you can also empower patients and caregivers to be their own advocates by being sensitive to the medical circumstances surrounding your patients' need for care. It is important for you to fully understand and grasp what led up to your patients' admission so that you may better understand the big picture and not make any preliminary judgements based on what is currently seen or written.

Do not hesitate to ask your patients questions beyond what is in their medical record to get a full understanding of their story. By the time you have seen your patient, reflect on how many people truly sat with them and asked them to fully share the events around such a vulnerable time in their lives.

By doing this, you are empowering the patient to unapologetically share what has transpired, and you are giving them the choice to voice their story. This will always give you a deeper understanding of your patients' needs than by simply reading through their medical record.

Empowering your patients is also listening to how they may be coping with their current situation. Many times, patients will come into your care feeling frustrated, angry, worried, and deeply concerned about their future health. In these circumstances, your patients are not necessarily looking for you to have all of the answers but to listen and validate the emotions such events have caused in their lives.

For instance, you might hear the frustration in your patients' voice from complaining about having to make repeat trips to the emergency room or to their family doctor until someone realized something was wrong. You might hear regret from your patients who waited too long to act on their concerns, hoping that their conditions would improve and that they wouldn't need your care to begin with.

Also, listen in to the patients who do not verbally express how they feel but, rather, visually appear sad, irritated, or worried. Even if you are incorrect in what you sense, it never hurts to ask them if there is something more going on that could be affecting their progress or participation.

Another valuable tool to empower patients and caregivers to be their own advocates is to be transparent and involving them in discharge planning as early as possible. Just as it is important to understand your patients' story preceding their need for care, it is just as important to discover where they want to be by the end of their course with you.

This will allow patients to understand the progressive nature of your care, that their progress will be incremental and not stagnant. It will also give your patients the idea that their success is dependent on their participation in all aspects of their care and not just yours. It will give them a sense of self-responsibility, accountability, and control over the direction of their lives from this point forward.

During my first two sessions with patients, I discuss the discharge goals and treatment plan to support their goals. Without discussing the end result, it would be a challenge to come up with a functionally directed treatment plan. For patients who cannot fathom that they can actually achieve what they want, then breaking down the end-goal to very short-term goals allows them to better ease into their program.

You might hear your patients say, "Never did I think I would make it to this point when I first came into your care." Or, "I never realized how hard it would be to walk again." Regardless of whether your patients achieve their goals, it allows them to gain perspective and insight into their needs.

Remember, your patients are not expected to know what to do or how to do it in order to get to where they desire to be. It has been my experience that patients either underestimate or overestimate the amount of time it takes to achieve a greater sense of function and independence.

By keeping your patients' goals at the forefront of every treatment, it gives them time to plan and determine if the goals need to be re-evaluated or are achievable. By being visible and transparent from the beginning, patients will feel they can rely on you to help them navigate through the system to receive the best care possible. In some cases, patients will start to look to you as an advocate of their care as well.

6

Focus on Solutions, not Barriers

As healthcare providers, we are mainly confronted with patients who have health challenges and problems. The focus of your work is to help your patients overcome these circumstances, while restoring hope and their ability to self-manage their health again. Since patients are coming to you with a change for the worse in their health status, you can imagine that their frame of mind would be negative.

This negative mindset is often the cumulative result of increased stressors, inability to cope, sudden onset of illness, and perceived lack of support. You may find your patients focusing on what they lack and on the barriers, hindering their possibility for success. Even the most motivated of patients will sometimes feel defeated, hopeless, and frustrated.

As a result, we are bombarded by many barriers for which our patients need help to overcome. One of your unique skills is to help your patients focus their energy on the different ways to achieve their health goals through and around those barriers. If you focus your patients' attention on their barriers, nothing will change, and you may only be instilling fear in them to act at all.

Shortly after my father's second liver transplant in February 2007, he suffered a major seizure and brain injury. The neurological team was then referred to his care, and, upon assessing him, they identified no neural activity. At this point, the neurology and transplant team held a brief conference with my mother, sister, and brother, strongly encouraging to take him off of life support.

My sister remembers a very big round-table meeting being held, with our family on one side and the medical teams on the other. While the neurology team was recommending taking my dad off of life support, my father's transplant surgeon—his "angel," as my mother referred to him—kept saying my dad needed more time to heal.

My sister vividly described my mother clenching her hands in front of the surgeon, pleading not to give up on my dad. With his advocacy and medical opinion, an understanding was arrived at with the neurology team to wait to see if anything changed over the weekend. If nothing changed, we would take my dad off of life support.

I remember walking into the conference room that day after school. They had just finished the meeting, and I witnessed my mother, sister, and brother wailing. They explained what had been said, and I began to bawl. We sat alone in the room for a while after the meeting, in periods of complete silence, wonder, and shock, to moments of hysterically mourning my father.

I vividly remember my mom telling each of us what my dad thought of us through her tears. She pointed to me: "You were the apple of his eye. He was always proud of you." Although I always felt that, hearing it made it all feel too real, and missing him was becoming my new reality.

We knew we did not want him to suffer, but we could not let him go just like that. We could not give up on him and give up for him. My dad always did what he wanted to do, and, if he wanted to die, he would have died. If he was being called to leave us, it would have happened for him. I truly felt, in the very core of my being, that decisions were all happening too prematurely.

As hope would have it, the very next day, my father started to show basic responses: blinking, squeezing hands, etc. The neurologist was called to reassess his neural activity, and, upon doing so, he stated, "This is remarkable…I have never seen anything like it." He was stunned and baffled, and implied that my dad's journey should be captured and documented. Perhaps he may have even been a little spiritually enlightened.

As you can imagine, our family became hopeful and optimistic. We cried but with tears of joy this time. However, my dad's time continued to pass in the hospital, and, in June, our family was once again called to a conference. This meeting was one of the worst—we were informed my dad would never breathe on his own, walk, talk, or eat again. The recommendation was discharge for long-term care with no chance of recovery. The only team member not at the table was his transplant surgeon.

I always found it interesting how he was never in favour of these doom-and-gloom meetings. His absence and solution-focused demeanor kept us hopeful. I also found it interesting how we never heard from all team members at once about their opinions on my dad's prognosis. There were several teams involved in my dad's care but never a comprehensive one.

We later discovered that his transplant surgeon still believed my dad just needed more time despite what was said at the meeting. He understood my dad's journey from the beginning, and, because he believed, so did we. Later that month, my dad was breathing on his own and transferred to the transplant unit and becoming more mobile. Can you imagine how we'd have felt—in hindsight—if we had taken him off of life support?

I do not believe my dad's surgeon necessarily expected my father to make a complete recovery, but I do know that he had the insight to focus on the solutions hidden deep within my dad's barriers, while the rest of the team was ready to dismiss any other options.

As a healthcare provider today, I respect him for going against the grain and defending the underdog in my dad. I deeply believe he would not have done so if he did not expect my father to eventually make it home. Despite all of his medical knowledge and expertise, he also knew how dedicated a family we were and knew my father's strong will to survive after all he had been through.

My father's primary solution was time, and, as progress was slowly seen, more time was needed. As a family, we witnessed his recovery unfolding, and it then became our mission to protect my dad's energy from any negativity or barriers. We had to transform our belief into faith in my dad's healing and recovery. Even if no one else believed, we had to. If we had not been so dedicated to his healing, no one else would have been.

Our faith served my dad and family during his journey. My parents are spiritual beings. We believe in higher reason, in God, and in miracles. My mother always carried and surrounded my dad with mementos—rosaries, prayers, saints, the Virgin Mary, Jesus, etc. We would place them all over his room, particularly around his bedside. They were on the bedrails, in his pillow cases, and pinned to his hospital gowns.

She was his biggest protector—spending 16 hours every day in the hospital with him. We heard more negative than positive when it came to my dad's prognosis, but we always believed in him until we found other professionals who would start to believe as well. Sometimes, our persistent belief gained the faith of other health professionals because a lot of his recovery could not be otherwise medically explained.

One year to the day after my father's transplants, he was discharged to our family home. He knew who we were, he recognized his house, and he was able to breathe, walk, talk, and eat on his own. He did have higher-level cognitive deficits that required us to help with banking, paying bills, housekeeping, and shopping. He no longer could drive, although he did try once and did so successfully. But even that shocked him, and he never drove again.

I'm not saying that the last 11 years of his life were not complicated, because they very much were, but he surpassed all the medical odds that were stacked against him over those 11 years. He truly was an underdog and a medical miracle.

One of my dad's first follow-up appointments was with his transplant team. I remember his team gathered around him, including his physiotherapist, who was so happy to see he was up and walking around with his two-wheeled walker. Another doctor poked his head through, asking, "Where is this Lazarus?" To them, he literally did arise from the dead, and it was heartwarming for them to witness this miracle with their own eyes.

I have learned through my dad's journey and those of some of my patients over the years that science cannot explain or predict everything. Sometimes we are struck with spontaneous forms of recovery and spontaneous forms of illness. Despite all of this, I hope that my dad's story inspires healthcare providers to always look beneath the surface of what they may not be able to see and be guided by what they truly believe.

Sometimes it is in the unexplainable that solutions are discovered. Time is a great example of this. While I understand our healthcare system can support our patients for only so long, it is our responsibility to ensure that patients do not get overlooked and are guided in how to continue following up on their care.

I encourage you to be a problem-solving provider who leads your patients by solutions and spirit. To focus on your patient's barriers is destructive; it will only create more problems and leave your patients or caregivers feeling hopeless and anguished. In my opinion and from my personal experience, unless you are without-a-doubt certain of your patient's prognosis, hope should never be taken off of the table.

This does not mean misleading patients, creating false hope, or telling them what they want to hear but, rather, being fully transparent and working with your patients to find safe solutions that could add more value to their life *in the moment*.

How to Focus on Solutions

In the initial stages, when patients are admitted into your care, they may feel overwhelmed, anxious, and lacking motivation. These feelings and emotions tend to be brought on by perceived barriers within and around them, such as their medical conditions, the institutions, multiple healthcare providers or teams, pain, medications, tests, schedules, etc.

One of the most valuable lessons I learned—first as a caregiver and then as a healthcare provider—is that there is always faith. A big part of my practice is encouraging patients to have faith in time and in the process of restoring wellness. All other barriers will be amplified if patients begin with a lack of faith and belief in themselves or their healthcare system.

Clearly let your patients know from the onset of assessment what you believe they can expect to achieve—at a minimum—during their time with you. This is based on clinical competency, experience, awareness, and sensitivity to others' needs. You will earn patients' faith and trust by sincerely practicing in their best interests every day, despite what challenges you may face from them or others.

Often times, when patients need your care, they are either very vague or very concrete about their goals. For instance, a patient whose primary complaint is pain might simply say, "I just want my back pain to go away." Or, a patient who has lost the ability to walk might say, "I just want to walk again."

Dig deeper into your patients' goals by asking what it would mean to them to be able to achieve these goals. These emotionally driven reasons will get them through the challenging phases of healing. Also, ask what it is they can do right now to move closer to full recovery. This will take their focus off what they do not have and put it more on what they actually want and can have.

If your role is one in which provider-patient interaction is limited and very short-term in nature, then it is recommended that you provide your patient with reasonable, short-term solutions as well as opportunities to explore their goals more closely by referring them to other healthcare providers or community resources.

The combination of short-term solutions and longer-term follow-up will give patients a greater understanding of the nature of their condition, the time they need, and relevant treatment options.

Furthermore, monitoring your patients' progress is essential to objectively outlining how they have improved during their time with you. It is difficult for some patients to reflect on their progress because they are so focused on that one big goal. Many times, that one big goal is an accumulation of smaller, successive goals. Accomplishment of these goals in themselves are also solutions and should be acknowledged and celebrated.

For example, if your patient has not walked in months, strive to first promote independence in bed mobility, positioning, or gentle stretching. This will build their confidence while working toward walking again.

Using outcome measures such as questionnaires or functional testing is a great visual tool for your patients to appreciate their progress. This will allow you to safely promote independence while minimizing risk to your patients.

For patients whose primary goal is to be pain-free, find the safest exercises and positions, and modify activities that reduce pain or create no added pain. After some time, repeat and compare their outcome measures to their first day. The positive change in status will empower your patients to feel like they are capable of regaining function and managing their pain. This all builds your patients' trust in you as their provider, and it motivates them to participate further in your plan.

Healthcare providers who are "solution-oriented" have the ability to lead patients to take action by focusing on what they can improve about their circumstances. While working in a hospital setting, the most common goal I work toward with my patients is returning home at a level where they can independently function within their own home. Yet, because of the nature of their condition, they may need assistance with even simpler tasks like repositioning themselves in bed or a chair.

It is my responsibility to share this insight and perspective with my patients. This refocuses my patients' outlook from "perfection" to "progression" and takes the burden off of them to feel that they need to be 100% before returning home again. My position is to facilitate my patients' functional growth, not restrict it. I do this by first helping them focus on being independent in a controlled hospital setting.

An example is restoring independence of getting in and out of the bed, or sitting and standing from a chair before walking independently. I do not think the majority of my patients expect to be quickly rehabilitated, however, I do believe they expect to have a reliable healthcare provider to help set them up for success as early as possible. Success is discovering another way for your patients to work on some aspect of their overall goal independently.

By also re-focusing your patients' attention to the present, you will help improve their spirit and calm their mind and body. Eventually, by introducing solutions systematically, your patients' progress will begin to unfold. As their healthcare provider, you can feel proud and reassured of your role when patients' belief in themselves starts to grow.

When my patients express to me before I even suggest to them, "I would like to try to walk to the bathroom myself now," or, "Let me try to lift my own legs in and out of bed," it demonstrates that they are feeling empowered to initiate the conversation around solutions and self-managing their health safely.

It further reinforces the realization in my patients that such a simple task is fundamental to going home and living more independently. And that is an accomplishment worth recognizing.

As patients start to appreciate that they have the ability to manage aspects of their care in the present state, they start to look forward to the next goal, the next big step. It is a privilege and our duty as their healthcare providers to see them through to the next goal safely.

The shift in focus to solutions will propel your patients forward, and you will notice your patients beginning to direct their care needs and be willingly involved in their goal setting.

Better health, improved function, and restored independence suddenly begin to feel like a reality, rather than just a possibility or memory.

After my father's transplant surgeries and subsequent brain injury, we knew his life was fragile. We knew we could lose him at any time. We also knew it was possible that he would never know who we were or how to live remotely independently again.

We were just desperately seeking a healthcare provider to have just enough faith in him and in time. If it were not for his surgeon, who encouraged us to focus on his slow-but-steady progress, he would have never survived. And as a result, my life and practice as a healthcare provider would probably look very different.

When my father eventually came home in 2008, he shared with us what he experienced during his second transplant surgery. He remembered hearing the voices of doctors, some saying, "Let him go...he isn't going to make it..." and then hearing one particular voice persisting: "We have to keep working." Sure enough, they did. It was the voice of an angel.

7

Create a Safe Therapeutic Environment

Creating a safe therapeutic environment for your patients, one in which your patients feel welcome, accepted, and eager to work with you, involves integrating a combination of the six previous strategies into your practice every day.

Earlier in my career, I took on a position in a clinic and was being oriented to my future caseload. During this time, I was observing some patient sessions among therapists, and one of the sessions had a profound impact on me.

In this particular situation, the therapist was working with an elderly man who had a language barrier. The patient had just recently had shoulder surgery, and they were working on regaining his range of motion.

Rehab following shoulder surgery can often be quite painful, however, this patient was nearly crying because he was in so much agony. I observed the therapist's lack of compassion toward him, and it seemed this was not the first time the patient had cried.

Professionally, I do not believe in the "no pain, no gain" philosophy. The patient's range of motion was quite limited, but perhaps it was not just because of his stiff shoulder, but because something was lacking in the rapport with his therapist to allow him to safely push through this critical phase of his treatment plan.

I can remember itching to work with the patient as soon as I could, because I wanted to try approaching him in a completely different manner. I truly believed making him feel safe in the therapeutic space would enable him to break through to the next level of his progress.

For one, I empathized with the patient because my parents are also immigrants, and I knew he just needed compassionate education, persistent encouragement, and gentle guidance to gain his trust. Although healthcare providers might understand the rationale behind our patients' pain and limited movements, patients cannot be expected to, and so, it warrants timely attention and explanation.

I also committed to listening to both his verbal and non-verbal expressions. In doing so, I could educate and reassure him on the normalcy surrounding his pain experience. I was then able to explain how we would safely manage his pain while demonstrating the exercises he would be doing to regain functional independence.

Most importantly, I continued to reassure him over the course of our sessions, and, although his progress was slower, he did achieve his goals. He and his wife were so grateful that they purchased coffee and donuts for the whole staff. This was a patient who went from feeling fearful, unsure, and in extreme pain, to feeling like he belonged and was enjoying independence again.

Similarly, in the same setting, I started working with a younger male, in his early 40s, and he explained to me how he was off work because of persistent neck pain. He appeared worried and anxious about how debilitated he was feeling. After asking questions about his history, I discovered he had seen other healthcare providers but was not improving.

He shared some of the previous treatments he had been receiving and he allowed me to assess his pain. After a thorough assessment, I did not see any red or yellow flags to indicate anything sinister. I explained to him that I recommended implementing a functional and active treatment plan, one in which he would ultimately be independent in carrying out while still managing his pain. I came to this conclusion based on his personal history around his injury and my findings, as well as the treatment from other providers. I felt there were gaps between his story and the treatment that had been implemented. To me, it was a no-brainer as to why he was not improving. However, to him, it was extremely complicated. I just needed him to trust me.

I further explained that his pain would be managed but also that it would not be the only focus of treatment. His function would be the focus. His goals of returning to an active lifestyle and to work would be the focus of what we worked towards.

I will never forget the panicked look he gave when I explained what was recommended. When I asked him what was going on, he expressed fear of more pain, the possibility of not achieving his goals, and letting pain control his life. After all of this time, nothing was changing, so why would it now?

He could not quite wrap his head around the concept, and I understood why. I listened, I reassured him, I educated him, and I asked for permission to treat his concerns. It was big for me to have gained his trust after all of his previous unsuccessful attempts.

After several weeks, I saw a whole new man. He appeared confident and had a hop in his step. He would sign into the clinic, grab his treatment record, and independently carry out his exercises to perfection. Pain was managed, but it was only a small part of his sessions. He went on to socializing with friends, renovating his home, and eventually returning to work.

He was grateful. He was liberated. He felt empowered that he was no longer controlled by pain because he knew how to manage it. He was more in tune with his body and was living life again. By allowing him to express his worry, validate his fears, ask questions, give permission, and be actively involved in his goals, I was able to create a safe environment for him to get his life back.

Creating a safe therapeutic environment for your patients means understanding that, despite their diagnosis, their needs remain unique. There are no two patients alike in this world. A chiropractor shared with me how she creates a safe space for her patients that supports their personal story as well as the emotional and physical aspects of their injuries.

She practices with open ears and a compassionate heart, as she listens with the intention to better understand her patients' exact concerns and experiences. She was recently met with a first-year college student who was complaining of right-side chest pressure and tension. The patient had first been cleared by his doctor as it was believed that his issues were muscle-related in nature.

Upon examining him, she did not find anything to be clinically producing his symptoms, yet she knew her patient was legitimately having pain. She made it a point to pull up a chair, sit next to him, and create a safe space for him to explain his concerns in more detail. Upon doing this, she discovered that her patient was finding school extremely stressful and that, around exam time, his pain would surface and debilitate him.

The chiropractor could empathize with her patients' issues, as they paralleled her own when she was a student. When the chiropractor shared this with the patient, he immediately showed a sense of relief. Finally, he was met with a healthcare provider who led with the genuine intent to help, above all else.

Once she was able to establish the root cause for her patients' concerns, he was able to fully engage in his care, and she was able to educate on tips and strategies to alleviate stress and anxiety. By the end of their session, her patient was laughing, smiling, and grateful.

The care she provided to her patient was intuitively sensed through her clinical assessment. She did not give up on him but, rather, allowed him to tell her more that could help her get to the root of his concerns. This opened the channels of communication for him to share his story and then receive the care she would be able to provide.

How to Create a Safe Therapeutic Environment

Creating a safe therapeutic environment means making your patients feel reassured and comfortable in your care throughout your interactions with them. Patients come to us because they trust that we have the knowledge and skills to treat their limitations. However, I believe patients *stay* with us because of our sensitivity and ability to understand the nature of their needs and seeing progress towards their goals.

First, when you have become aware of new patients in your space, it is thoughtful to approach them and ask for their permission to introduce yourself and explain your role in upcoming sessions together. By first asking for permission, you are empowering the patient to be in control of their personal space in the greater clinical environment.

In the hospital setting, patients who are admitted onto an inpatient unit are often out of sorts and are feeling furthest from themselves. They are still processing how they came to be in this space, unfamiliar to their everyday life. They essentially have no privacy, as they are met with roommates and staff walking in and out of their room multiple times a day.

In an outpatient setting, some patients may grow anxious waiting to be called into your session. They may also feel like they are one of many who need care and are uncertain of how you can help and understand them out of the dozens of patients you met with today. They may feel that you do not have enough time. Upon interacting with them, you may notice they are anxious or rushed in sharing their concerns.

In situations such as these, make it a point to appear calm and unrushed. Your patients will mirror your own mannerisms. If you are high strung and feel pressed, you might provoke that in your patient, who is likely already anxious about their issues. This is not the type of environment that facilitates focused healing and recovery.

Yet, if you take the time to smile, sit down at your patients' level, embody a safe space for discussion, and do not look at your watch or the clock, you will create an atmosphere that is peaceful and unrestricted by outside barriers.

It also helps to ask if there is anything you can do to make your patients feel more comfortable, such as offering water or opening/closing the blinds. This ensures them that this is their space now and that you are focused on making their time with you valuable and productive.

The best approach is to make your presence about your patients and not about you. By simply showing up, human-to-human, you are allowing your patients to connect with themselves in this unfamiliar space. This will allow them to feel at ease and reassured that you are eager to help them so that they may build their trust in you and their team.

Allow patients the time to share their story and for you to tune into their concerns. This will open the channels of communication between you and your patients. When your patients enter your space, as new as it may be, transitioning into care will be easier if they feel safe to ask questions, express their concerns, and proclaim their goals without judgement.

Furthermore, if patients feel they are free to be themselves, they will be more open to your clinical reasoning and recommendations for their plan of care. In this openness, they will be more likely to offer additional information rather than withhold it. The more information patients are able to give you, the more effective and individualized your treatments will be.

When interacting with your patients, pay attention to your energy, your words, and your expressions. Some patients' conditions can be challenging. Do your patients leave feeling productive, motivated, and hopeful? Do they feel heard and assured? Do they feel you took the time to listen and follow up on their concerns? Do they trust that you have their best interests at heart? Regardless of what you have to share, there is always a safe and tactful way to express it and leave your patients feeling like you genuinely care.

Creating a safe therapeutic space also involves the physical environment you surround your patients with in every session. Physically creating a safe space means the environment and equipment are safely kept and attended to. It also includes having a minimum level of clinical competency that reassures patients will be safe in your hands—literally, in some cases.

If you have tuned in enough to your patients and know that certain environmental factors will help improve their mood and participation, you should definitely implement them. For instance, some patients enjoy music, while others do not. Some patients may feel more relaxed in a dim setting; some may feel more energized by brighter lighting. Some patients focus better when the space is busy, while some focus better when it is quiet and serene. Some patients feel more comfortable with their friends or family present, while some patients specifically request no one else attend their visits.

Essentially, take the time to ask your patients what they prefer, and do your best to tailor the treatment space to support their recovery. Tuning into their needs will optimize their healing, satisfaction, and sense of importance. One healthcare provider takes the time to write inspiring quotes and wellness tips in her treatment room each week based on the common concerns or issues her clients have been working through.

Create a safe space between you and your patients that is professional yet respectful of their dignity and confidentiality. In my experience, some patients may downplay their entitlement of dignity when they are in a healthcare provider's environment. Perhaps their vulnerability makes them feel the need to surrender and have no control over their care. Make it a point to redirect them in their belief, and inspire dignity by providing care that makes them feel at ease and in control.

As healthcare providers, our own physical positioning and posturing when providing care speaks for itself. Despite how your patients may be feeling, there should be something about your presence that gives them hope and minimizes fear. If you are uncertain or hesitant, your patients will feel insecure and at risk. If you are confident in your competency and in your gifts, your patients will sense this and will be more apt to place their trust in you.

Providing care to your patient outside of direct clinical care also fosters a safe therapeutic space. This shows itself in those small-but-mighty details throughout a patient's day that allow it to flow just a little more smoothly. You can help patients plug their cell phones or tablets into the wall charger above their hospital bed. You can take the time to read a consent form or questionnaire to patients who are unable to read and ensure that they understand before you proceed.

Take the time to go beyond what is expected of you in such a way that is not grandiose but ordinary and helpful. This is not only providing good care; it is also just being a good person. These are the small things that go into creating the best patient experience. When patients are offering reviews by the end of their time with you, it is the reviews around their direct care that mean just as much as the care itself.

Prevent Unnecessary Conflict

O nce you have developed a deeper understanding of your patient as a whole person, you will become more intuitive and adaptable to their unique characteristics. You will begin to appreciate the non-physical qualities about them that need your understanding and attention in order to guide them through a successful course of treatments with you.

I have worked with many patients over the years who do not like change and have regimented personalities. I have also worked with many patients who are extremely laid-back and did not take their own concerns as seriously as I did. I have worked with patients who are even a combination of the two in some way. The point is, lead with what your patients convey is important to them.

Sometimes what matters most to your patients is unexpressed verbally, so it is important to pay close attention and note why they may not be responding fully to your care. When you have been seeing your patients regularly and have developed rapport, you may notice something is off with them on a particular day. It is acceptable and appropriate to ask what is on their mind and point out the change you are noticing. This further reinforces your patients' sense of importance.

I can recall a patient of mine with whom I'd been working regularly showing up to his session one day in poor spirits. Although he consented to treatment and felt fine to participate, he was limited by something I could not see. I made him aware of his unusual demeanor, and he suddenly started venting about his "off morning." He was accustomed to his morning routine, and when staff were not exactly on his schedule, it really threw him off for the rest of his day.

Because he was able to share how he felt and reveal his perspective, I was able to listen and validate his concerns. In doing so, he became more receptive to me offering insight from a staff member's perspective. I also ensured I would communicate his concern with staff so that we could all come to a working agreement. His mood immediately improved, and he was able to resume his session as per his usual pleasant self. The issue never surfaced again.

As healthcare providers, we have an intuitive gift of knowing when our patients are being authentic or not. We also have the gift of connecting, and, so, if you are unsure why your patients are not responding favorably to your care, simply ask them. Oftentimes, their response has nothing to do with you, and they truly do want to work with you towards their goals, but, instead, something else is on their mind. By asking them, you may be able to help them and maybe even prevent a potential conflict in the near future.

In most cases, knowing what is important to your patients is what will allow them to fully participate in your care. Once you are able to identify the goals or aspects of care that mean the most to your patients, that is the best place to begin implementing care. For many patients, what matters most is a basic level of functioning that has been taken away from them.

If you have been truly engaged with your patients, you will come to understand that it is not only the care itself you provide that matters but also the way in which it is provided. Are you courteous? Are you being transparent? Are you creating an environment that tends to their preferences? Are you scheduling your patients in such a way that it optimizes their chances of success?

Lack of communication or miscommunication is one of the biggest causes of patient complaints and medical errors in the healthcare system. When you're working on an inpatient hospital unit, it's easy to take for granted the fact that patients are staying for a prolonged period of time.

As a result, we may think they would be more understanding of adapting to changes in our schedule to meet the needs of all patients. Yet, what we may fail to recognize is that our patients want us to treat them as individuals—not necessarily as a collective entity. All patients have an individual goal, and they want to get the most out of their time with you to bring them closer and closer to their foreseeable outcomes.

I have learned over the years that *because* patients are living in hospital, they are entitled to and need notice of any changes in their care schedule. Many patients actually appreciate the upfront communication, and, in turn, they will accept and will fully participate in the treatment plans. However, if they are caught off guard and without reasonable explanation or apology, it can cause unnecessary disappointment.

In an outpatient setting, when changes need to be made to patients' schedules, simply giving them enough notice of the change will save you a lot of damage control in the long run, and patients will continue to work openly with you.

Additionally, in an outpatient setting, you may not be seeing your patients as frequently as you would in an inpatient setting. In such cases, it is important to ensure patients feel that you are managing their care concerns with utmost importance either directly, by referral, or by appropriate follow-up. Amidst all of your patients, your intention should be to treat the one patient in your presence in that moment.

Once my dad returned home in 2008, he received home-care services daily to support his self-care needs. The organization providing care tried its best to maintain a continuity of healthcare providers and, for the most part, was great at doing so. It came as a surprise when one of his support workers who provided care left him unattended afterward, when my mother was not home.

The healthcare provider knew my dad was unable to mobilize independently and would be a high fall risk. Yet, after helping him to get ready for bed, he left the home, believing that he would fall asleep. Thankfully, my father was safe, but you can imagine my and my mother's anxiety when we came home to see my dad sitting up bright-eyed in bed, slightly confused by our panicked concern.

Although the healthcare provider had acted with good intent, had my father fallen out of bed or while trying to stand on his own, it could have resulted in serious injury or harm. It would have been safer if he had just waited for my mother, as he expected her to return within the hour, rather than rushing to the next client. Situations like these are just not worth the risk to your patients' health and to creating a conflict that was completely avoidable.

How to Prevent Unnecessary Conflict

One of the best ways you can prevent potential conflict is to understand that it will inevitably happen. It can happen internally, within yourself, or externally, among others and your environment. By simply understanding that conflict comes with the great responsibility of being a healthcare provider, you will be more likely to work through it more constructively.

If conflict arises in your workplace and among team members, it is important to empathize with one another to come to a workable resolution. At the end of the day, we have more in common with each other than we are different. We have a passion to serve others. We spend more time with each other than we do with our loved ones, and we are all trying to find our place in this thing called "work" that enables us to love what we do every day.

So, if your co-worker is having an off-day or acting out of character, kindly ask if they are alright. In the same scenario, if your co-worker is being unkind toward you, ask if they are alright. Like your patients, chances are if your colleagues are not acting like themselves, it has nothing to do with you and everything to do with how they are processing the feelings of an event that might have happened in their lives.

In exceptional circumstances of conflict where reaching out to your colleague is beyond your control, it would be appropriate to seek counsel from someone you can trust within your organization.

It is important to feel like you can find compassion and sanctuary in your colleagues in order to deal with the ups and downs of every working day. I have been in toxic working environments that I tried to avoid and minimize by focusing on providing the best patient care possible. However, these suppressed feelings still affected my sense of satisfaction, value, and belonging. I now realize that, in order for our patients to have the greatest care experience, we have to first feel like we work in an environment that brings out the best in us.

You are also responsible for the energy and efforts you bring to your workplace every day. Although it is not your job to secure others' happiness, it is your responsibility not to let your personal conflicts affect the overall team connection and atmosphere.

Internal conflict is the kind in which you may find yourself almost daily. That internal dialogue goes on constantly in the background of your mind as you are trying to complete your day-to-day tasks with competency and fulfilment.

Everyone deals with internal conflict differently. For many healthcare providers, ethical dilemmas are a common cause of internal conflict. I prefer to bounce thoughts and feelings off of trusted team members to gain clarity, while some prefer to keep to themselves and work through it quietly. Either way, internal conflict is more about you as a person and a healthcare provider than it is about what is going on around you.

In order to understand the work environment we find ourselves in every day, we have to better understand ourselves. In reference to Chapter 1, once you have defined your personal purpose, your working purpose becomes merely an extension of it. Rather than conform to a system that does not support your purpose, you can create one or find one that does. The realization that your purpose is priceless will bring you fulfilment every day.

Another way to prevent potential conflict is to plan for it. Planning for conflict does not mean creating it, expecting the worst, or acting out of fear, but it means to lead with the best interests and values of your patients first. If you know that your patients value transparency and being fully informed of every aspect of their care, you would do your best to be visible, follow up regularly, and communicate with their health team to provide a comprehensive experience.

You may come to find through your interactions with patients that they often lack confidence, not only in themselves but also in the healthcare system as a whole. Along the way in their health journey, perhaps they were misinformed or left unaware of circumstances surrounding their care. You can prevent unnecessary conflict by communicating directly with your patient about their care as often as they need.

In the event you cannot answer their questions or share certain information, make it your responsibility to find someone who can. Appreciate that your patients trust you to do right by them, otherwise, they would not ask for your help. The greatest peace of mind for your patient is knowing that you have done all you can for them during their time with you. In turn, this is also your greatest peace of mind—knowing you have done your best and all that you could for your patients.

While conflict is common among healthcare providers and in the healthcare system, unnecessary conflict arises when a negative situation occurs that was preventable and avoidable. These generally stem from very small-scale and unnoticed matters that can manifest into a greater web of concern and conflict.

I like to think of unnecessary conflict as communication that has fallen through the cracks. Unnecessary conflict is deeply rooted in a lack of reliable communication systems, mainly collective purpose and shared empathy.

Imagine you are a physiotherapist working in a clinic, and a patient came to you after an ankle fracture to begin therapeutic exercise. The patient comes empty-handed without a physician's order or script but is confident he is able to begin rehab per his doctor's verbal orders.

You need to know if he is able to weight-bear on his foot before you implement any weight-bearing exercises. The patient *seems* cognitively intact; do you take his word for it, or do you contact the physician directly?

You explain your conflict to your patient, and, although he tells you it is fine to weight-bear, something in you tells you to contact the physician directly for confirmation. You explain to your patient you do not want to cause unnecessary harm to his healing and would rather confirm with the physician.

Your patient understands and is agreeable. Upon calling the doctor, you receive confirmation that he is able to weight-bear only 25% or less on that leg. You have completely prevented the unnecessary harm that could have occurred had you listened to your patient's motivated attitude yet incorrect interpretation.

As your patient's therapist, you remained committed to your purpose of minimizing risk to helping your patient and empathizing with his desire to restore his function. In doing so, you realized by simply investing minimal time to call for clarification from the doctor, it could have a significant impact on his level of care and safety. Although your patient hoped his rehab course would have been quicker in nature, he would ultimately be grateful that you took the time to be thorough on his behalf.

You can also prevent unnecessary conflict by leading with good intention and integrity rather than out of fear or avoidance. I have learned over the years that dealing with conflict before you see it coming, just as you see it coming, or once it has arrived is better than avoiding it and hoping it will dissolve. Especially in an environment where there are many team members involved, it is very easy to defer or expect conflict to be handled by someone else.

If you are leading with kindness and willingness to do right by you, your patients, and your peers, it is easier to constructively manage conflict. However, if you are leading with defensiveness, hostility, or unwillingness to understand, you will come to find that conflict follows you. Ask yourself what is more important: to be right or to be understood? Conflict often arises from a misunderstanding—if we fail to come together to mutually understand the misunderstanding, the conflict will continue to resurface.

Conflict can also be a sign of professional awareness and growth. There is always something new to be learned, even in the most minor of incidences. If you can cope with conflict as a growth challenge, it will not paralyze you but, rather, shape you into a better healthcare provider and human being.

9

Reflect and Grow with Impact

Throughout your journey as a healthcare provider, it is only wise to continuously circle back to your purpose and reflect regularly on your practice. Your purpose serves as a marker or target that you are trying to obtain throughout the ebbs and flows of your career. It does not matter if the tides are high or low, slow or fast. The question is, "Did I do it all with purpose?"

As healthcare providers, we have to meet a minimum requirement of continuing education in order to better assess and treat our patients. Participation in clinical courses is essentially a form of reflection of wanting to improve a particular aspect of your practice.

However, I also believe that if we reflected more inward as our outward experiences grow, we can further improve our overall ability to care for our patients and bring fulfillment to our own lives. By reflecting on yourself in some capacity each and every day, the attitudes and skills you bring to your patients would be more positive and effective.

It is easier to focus on the negative occurrences that come with the high stress of changing people's lives every day. It is easier to get wrapped up in conflict resolution than in proud recognition of what was done successfully. Perhaps this is because it is expected of you to do good work and improve people's lives. But the reverse is also true: because you do good work and improve people's lives, it should be recognized and celebrated.

And so, until you reflect on the good with the poor, the happy with the sad, and the growth with the challenges, it will be difficult to focus on the overall abilities that you bring to your work every day. Even deeper, it is important to focus on these aspects of your personal life as well. Your work stems from who you believe you are, and who you are makes up those gifts you bring to your profession.

If you lack belief in yourself as a healthcare provider, then that will be reflected in how you care for your patients. Your uncertainty will show itself not only in your skills but in how you communicate with others. If belief is what you lack, then belief is what you need to reflect on, to ground yourself in your work.

It is only through self-reflection that you can gather your thoughts, feelings, reasonings, and commitments that will enable you to evolve into a better healthcare provider than you were yesterday. This will allow you to take pride in what you did well, learn from any mistakes, and consider how you could have done things differently.

Self-reflection is a practice of self-care. It is meant for you to discover what you are capable of and realize your potential as a healthcare provider. It is your way of acknowledging that what you do every day matters because what you do has an effect on your patients and on yourself.

Bringing more clarity to yourself will help you bring more clarity to your patients and team members. This puts you in a position to see every side, explain things clearly, listen openly, and ensure patients' safety. Self-reflection has no limits or conditions, so long as it brings your practice and purpose to another level of contentment.

As a caregiver, I often wondered if other healthcare providers reflected on their practice. During the many challenges we were faced with as a family advocating for my father, I would wonder if some healthcare providers really saw themselves or if they had just lost themselves. I would wonder if they felt fulfiled or if they felt compelled to do a job. It is one thing to do your job, but it is a whole other thing to do your job with grace, passion, and purpose.

It is no secret that, in order for you to last in the healthcare profession, you have to have a genuine love for humanity. I would often reflect on this, being the introvert that I am. To me, it always seemed counterintuitive—how am I able to create a strong therapeutic connection with my patients when the thought of interaction in its most basic form can make me feel uneasy?

The creation of this book is a complete, shared self-reflection. I have always said that "I am an introvert with an extroverted love for humanity." I have come to find that where my introversion excels is in leading my patients to solutions to improve their function, health, and well-being.

As an introvert, I seek meaningful connections, and there is nothing more meaningful than having the opportunity to help transform someone's life. When I am in such a space, my ability to communicate becomes more creative, authentic, and passionate. By working in purpose, I speak from my heart, and that is a language that everyone can connect with.

How to Reflect

First, applaud yourself for recognizing that there is always room to grow as a healthcare provider and as an individual. The thought of professional growth should trigger feelings of excitement, possibility, and clarity. If it triggers drained feelings of "more work," then this is not for you. Or, perhaps just not right now. And if not ever, then that's okay—it's not for everyone.

Second, applaud yourself for recognizing that you do not understand everything and that you can bring so much more to the table for your patients through learned experiences. If you are an entry-level provider, appreciate that you are not expected to know more than you know but, rather, show desire to stand on the shoulders of healthcare providers you respect and discover all that you can.

Third, do not overwhelm yourself by reflecting on all of the events of your day. Instead, reflect on one event that went well and one that was challenging. Acknowledge how each made you feel and why they may have surfaced to begin with. Reflect on what you would have changed and what you would not have changed about each situation.

Finally, reflect on how these situations have helped you evolve as a professional and on how bringing them to the surface in your mind will help you serve your next patient. If you are an experienced healthcare provider, ask yourself what has kept you here all these years. If you are a novice, ask yourself what has brought you here and what you want your future practice to look like.

We all become healthcare providers for the innate desire to help others, but as you jump in eagerly, you start to notice all of the technicalities surrounding care. That once-whispering voice, that once-fire in your soul, and that once-extra beat in your heart will be challenged by these circumstances.

You will have moments of despair, moments of self-doubt, moments of frustration, and moments of burnout. Feel all of it, reflect on it, but do not live in it. Do not bring it to your patients' experiences. Move beyond it. Remember, you have been called for something bigger, and there is no perceived barrier that can put out your spark. You revolutionize people's lives. That is where you live. That is who you are.

A Profound Reflection

My dad was our "Lazarus," as referred to by one of his transplant doctors when he returned home one year after his transplants. In my 11 years of practice, I find inspiration from my dad's stories of overcoming barriers, his strong will to live, and finding hope in a new day.

I am also inspired by my family, as we were so deeply involved in my dad's care, and by mom, who remained so dedicated and loving through it all. To this day, health professionals cannot explain how he recovered enough to know his family, return to his home, and learn how to eat, walk, and talk again. His recovery was referred to as a "spiritual miracle" by physicians and medical providers.

Although my dad came home for good in 2008, he was chronically ill and required caregiver support from my mother and me. He suffered a bowel obstruction, multiple debilitating seizures, chronic pneumonias, and other numerous infections.

As such, my dad had been in and out of hospitals, literally climbing out of bed, to try to go back home. He never spent an hour longer than he needed to. He would often scream at ambulance attendants not to take him to the hospital after falling ill at home.

He dreaded it. We dreaded it. We lived in fear of celebrating his better moments, knowing a decline in health would soon follow. Over time, we learned to be grateful for every lucid moment, wide smile, shared car ride, witty comment, intuitive insight, and loving remark.

On May 1, 2018, my father went to the hospital one last time. He had been admitted with infection, lack of appetite, and general weakness. I had spent that day with him and my mom, just as it always had been.

This time, he was not his usual spunky and resistant self. He was calm, finding comfort in his hospital bed, and tired. He had no energy to charm and give the staff a hard time when they were providing care. My mom never thought anything of it, as he'd always defied the odds; she believed he would come home again.

The provider in me knew medically his body was failing to thrive, and the daughter in me knew that he was too tired to fight anymore. Knowing my father did not like being in the hospital, I spent the day planning with community co-ordinators and the medical staff to arrange for my father to come home safely.

My mother was always by my dad's side when in hospital, and if she wasn't, one of us was, to support and care for him. My mother wanted to go to her cousin's funeral that evening, and I was to stay with him while she was gone.

In the past, when my mom would leave my dad's bedside to grab a coffee or quickly eat something, he would question her—asking where she was going and when she would be back. Sometimes he was joking, but, most times, it was his way of saying he needed her.

He depended on her, as he could not express or direct his care to hospital staff. They also relished each other's company, even in silence. He always wanted her nearby, as her loving nature protected him and gave him strength.

Shortly after my mom left for the funeral, I noticed a change in my dad's breathing. It was more laboured. The staff was not concerned initially. They allowed me to check his oxygen levels, and, although they appeared fine, he was not really responding. I also noticed a red rash on his lower leg that was starting to spread.

I called his nurse to reassess him, and she noticed the vascularity in his legs was changing. Her look of concern reinforced what I already knew—my dad was declining; it was likely that he was developing another infection. She contacted the doctor, but IV antibiotics were not an option, as my dad literally had no more accessible veins in his body. Not one single vein.

I immediately called my family; some of my siblings were already on their way, as we rotated visits throughout my dad's hospital stays. He was never alone. I explained what was happening to everyone as best as I could. My mom still did not believe it to be true—dad was slipping, for good. I called it before any of his providers did, unlike the umpteen times over the past 11 years. And it was killing me.

I comforted my dad, talked to him like I always had. Told him not to be afraid and if he were being called to go, we would be okay. When everyone had arrived, we all sat around his bedside, I rested my hand on his chest so as to calm his breathing. We prayed, called out for him, letting him know we were all there by his side. He shed multiple tears throughout his transition as his eyes remained open and fixated for hours. His spirit was very much present, and we all felt it.

Finally, at 2:45 a.m. on May 2, 2018, my dad took his last breath, and he closed his eyes peacefully. For all of the medical complications he'd endured over the years, his passing could not have been more beautiful. He was no longer in pain, and he was finally free. Free of falls, free of wheelchairs and canes, free of medications, free of infections, free of seizures, free of hospitals, and free of fear.

I often think back to that moment—that moment when he slipped as my mother left his bedside that day. That feeling, that memory has overpowered in ways that have knocked me to my knees. Why did he slip when it was just he and I?

I believe my dad trusted me to keep him safe and reassured. He knew I would not panic and that I would understand. I always looked after his medical care, and he knew that I knew that it was too much for him to bear.

He left us after giving every single vein in his body. He left me with the faith to believe in every underdog, those who have been struck by illness with no perceived medical chance of recovery, to rise again. Just like he did. My Lazarus.

Thank you, dad. As your youngest child, you always worried about me in life. Yet, I know for certain that your loving spirit surrounds me now and will never leave my side. Your struggles inspired the strength within me to write my truth and share it with the world. I know you are smiling down on me now. I miss your charismatic smile more than I could ever have imagined.

Thank you to every one of my patients who have trusted me to provide care in your time of need and in your pursuit of triumph. Thank you for letting me in and guiding you through to the next chapter of your life—one that I hope is filled with good health, peace, and bliss.

Thank you to my readers, encouragers, and supporters. Thank you for stepping into my world, looking out through my eyes, and feeling with my heart. Thank you for being in this, together.

Shared Reflections

"We, as professionals, can never assume to know our patients' truth or true story—even if we feel we have seen a similar scenario or heard a similar story before. Each is unique and deserves that we listen."

—Dijana Panzalovich, Occupational Therapist

"Effective communication is when you can patiently sit and listen to a patient with your heart, eyes, and ears. It is focused and non-judgemental, wide open, without any interruption. This will yield a deeper understanding in the implementation of a treatment plan."

—Dr. Natalie Cervini, Chiropractor

"If you take the time to listen, you can learn a lot from your patients. As told by a patient to me: 'You have a career and not a job. A job is from 9 to 5 and for a paycheck. A career has meaning and purpose.'"

—Lidia D'Alimonte, Physiotherapist

"In my experience, I've found the most important point in the nurse-patient relationship is at the very beginning, when building rapport. Listening and acknowledging from the start and being compassionate and honest helps patients to feel supported during difficult times such as hospitalization. It builds a strong, trusting relationship and may sometimes help lessen the anxieties many patients experience."

—Mary-Anne Konopasky, Registered Nurse

"I am all about being connected with clients individually and on their own level. My heart in what I do is huge in motivating and inspiring people to do their best and to be themselves. People will never forget how you made them feel. A small gesture of this kind often makes the biggest difference."

—Suzie Vidinovski, SueSanity Fitness

"I give patients the tools and strategies to empower themselves. I can give them suggestions for solving their problems, but they have to be empowered to make their own destiny in the end."

—Carla Milevski, Social Worker

"With regard to my career, if I ever stop being kind to the patients and families I am supporting, then it is time for me to retire or find another area of work. It is so important to remember our patients are going through some very challenging times and don't need someone with attitude or negativity making things more difficult."

—Carla Milevski, Social Worker

"Everyone has a story. The innate desire to share our experiences is the essence of our being at any age, developmental level, or physical/cognitive capacity. The ability to communicate comes in various forms. The communication continuum is vast and extraordinary. Eye gaze, gesture, physical movement, sign, voice, symbols, pictures, text, braille...whatever the manner, providing individuals with a venue to express themselves is an incredible process and an absolute privilege."

—Paula S. LaSala-Filangeri, Speech-Language Pathologist

"Communicating with patients is the best tool. Humour, respect, and trust are small gestures that can go a long way. A smile and kindness don't cost you anything but get you a lot. I learned about compassionate communication years ago from a dear colleague of mine who reminded me that we can pick up good qualities from amazing people."

—Gwen McAllen, Registered Practical Nurse

Your Reflections

i)   Why do you do what you do?

ii)   Who do you want to become as you journey through your career?

iii)   What area do you feel you excel in and bring the best care to your patients?

iv)   What area do you want to improve upon to bring the best care to your patients?

v)   Reflect on a situation that challenged your purpose. How did it challenge you? How did it shape who you are and the spirit with which you practice today?

vi)   Reflect on a time where being compassionately empathetic to your patient changed the course of your patient's progress. How did it make you feel?

vii)   Reflect on ways you could better listen to your patients. Reflect on the ways you currently find effective.

viii)   Reflect on that one moment when you gained the faith and belief of your colleagues or employers because you practiced in accordance with your moral code of conduct.

ix) In what ways do you empower patients and their caregivers to be their own advocates of care?

x) In what ways do you help your patients stay focused on solutions to achieve their goals?

xi) How do you create a safe therapeutic environment for your patients?

xii) Reflect on a time in your practice when you prevented an unnecessary conflict from happening because you saw it coming first.

xiii) Reflect on a case over the years that moved you, validated your purpose, and gave deeper meaning to your practice.

References

Anna Raberus, Inger K Holmstrom, Kathleen Galvin, Annelie J Sundler; The nature of patient complaints: a resource for healthcare improvements, *International Journal for Quality in Health Care,* mzy215, https://doi.org/10.1093/intqhc/mzy215

Chayer, C., Freedman, M. 2001. Frontal Lobe Functions. Curr Neurol Neurosci Rep (6): 547–52.

Hall LH, Johnson J, Watt I, Tsipa A, O'Connor DB (2016) Healthcare Staff Wellbeing, Burnout, and Patient Safety: A Systematic Review. PLOS ONE 11(7): e0159015.https://doi.org/10.1371/journal.pone.0159015

Healthcare Compliance Pros. 2018. Integrity: More than Just a Piece of the Healthcare Compliance Puzzle. http://www.healthcarecompliancepros.com/blog/integrity-more-than-just-a-piece-of-the-healthcare-compliance-puzzle-2/

Reader TW, Gillespie A, Roberts J. Patient complaints in healthcare systems: a systematic review and coding taxonomy. *BMJ Qual Saf* 2014;23:678-689

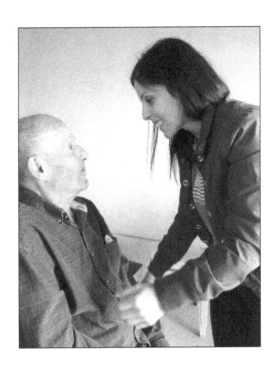

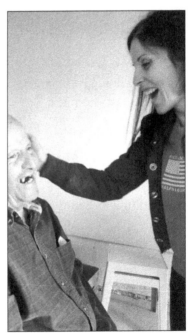

Dad (Jimmy George) and Jennifer 2016

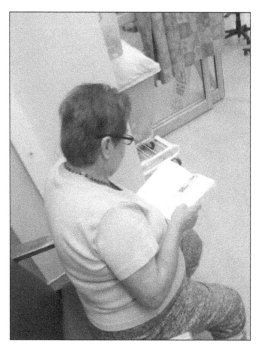

Margaret George, Jimmy's wife, praying in his
hospital room for his recovery (2007)

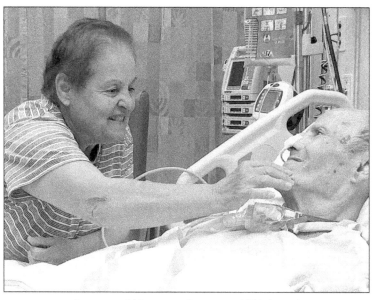

Jimmy and Margaret George in ICU (2007)

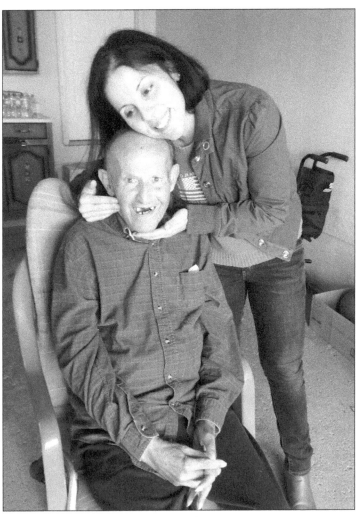

Jimmy George and Jennifer, in his favorite
room of the house, the garage (2016)